Y0-BWZ-665

Containing Health Benefit Costs:
The Self-Insurance Option

WITH CONTRIBUTIONS BY

William J. Bicknell, M.D.
Boston University Center for Industry
and Health Care and United Mine
Workers of America Health and
Retirement Funds

Jack H. Bleuler
Mobil Oil Corporation

John D. Blum
Boston University Center for Industry
and Health Care

Stephen C. Caulfield
United Mine Workers of America
Health and Retirement Funds

Richard H. Egdahl, M.D.
Boston University Center for Industry
and Health Care

Galt Grant
Polaroid Corporation

Michael J. Gulotta
American Telephone and Telegraph
Company

Donald P. Harrington
American Telephone and Telegraph
Company

Samuel X. Kaplan
United States Administrators

Brant Kelch
United Mine Workers of America
Health and Retirement Funds

William Michelson
United Storeworkers Security Plan

Robert B. Peters
Mobil Oil Corporation

Lesley L. Ralson
The Prudential Insurance Company of
America

Steven Sieverts
Blue Cross-Blue Shield of Greater New
York

Kevin Stokeld
Deere and Company

Richard W. Stone, M.D.
American Telephone and Telegraph
Company

Eleanor J. Tilson
United Storeworkers Security Plan

Diana Chapman Walsh
Boston University Center for Industry
and Health Care

David H. Winkworth
Mobil Oil Corporation

INDUSTRY AND HEALTH CARE 6

Containing Health Benefit Costs: The Self-Insurance Option

Edited by
Richard H. Egdahl and Diana Chapman Walsh

Springer-Verlag New York

Springer Series on Industry and Health Care
Richard H. Egdahl, M.D., PhD.
Diana Chapman Walsh, M.S.
Center for Industry and Health Care
Boston University Health Policy Institute
53 Bay State Road
Boston, Massachusetts 02215

Springer-Verlag New York Inc.
175 Fifth Avenue
New York, New York 10010

Library of Congress Cataloging in Publication Data
Main entry under title:

Containing health benefit costs.

(Industry and health care; 6)
    1. Insurance, Health—United States—Congresses.   I. Egdahl, Richard Harrison.   II.
Walsh, Diana Chapman.
HD7102.U4C62   338.4'3   79-156

All rights reserved.

No part of this book may be translated or reproduced in any form without written
permission from Springer-Verlag.

Copyright © 1979 by Springer-Verlag New York Inc.

Printed in the United States of America.

9 8 7 6 5 4 3 2 1

ISBN 0-387-90385-2 Springer-Verlag New York Heidelberg Berlin
ISBN 3-540-90385-2 Springer-Verlag Berlin Heidelberg New York

Preface

The springboard for this sixth volume in the Industry and Health Care series was a conference sponsored by the Center for Industry and Health Care of Boston University on June 9 and 10, 1978. That conference had a gradual genesis. Over a year ago we spent some time with Kevin Stokeld of Deere and Company and heard his views on self-insurance and self-administration as one device for a corporation to achieve better management control of its health benefit. More recent discussions with representatives of American Telephone and Telegraph Company and other corporations made it increasingly clear to us that management's need for data to monitor the use of employee health benefits was emerging as a critical policy issue. Subsequent meetings with executives at John Hancock Mutual Life Insurance Company in Boston and Mobil Oil Corporation in New York, among others, convinced us that simple answers would be elusive or inadequate and that there was a need for an objective and careful look at the evolving relationships between employee health benefits, claims administration, health services utilization, and corporate health care cost containment programs.

Since self-funding and particularly self-administration represent a fundamental change in the traditional insurance relationship, the conference was convened to explore the advantages and disadvantages of self-insurance for employee health benefits, with some attention to claims production but with special emphasis on the originating question of data for effective management of an employee health benefit. Background papers were prepared for the conference and distributed in advance to establish a common frame of reference and a basis for discussion. Most of the papers, in edited form, are included in this volume. Because Kevin Stokeld was unable to attend the conference, we arranged in advance to videotape an interview with him and opened the meeting with it. The Deere and Company chapter in this volume is an adaptation of that interview. The remainder of the meeting consisted of a day-and-a-half of give-and-take discussion between people representing the principal purchasers of group health insurance—business and the government—several of the major carriers, and other third-party administrators. Part I of this volume draws heavily on the dialogue, and, like the conference, seeks to elaborate the varying and sometimes divergent themes that arise in a wide-ranging discussion on the general topic of self-insurance.

We owe a special debt of gratitude to William J. Bicknell and to Kevin Stokeld, for valuable guidance and help during the period when the conference was being planned, and for their particularly important contributions to the conference and the book. We are grateful, as well, to the other authors of background papers, and also to the participants in the conference, whose reflections constitute the heart of Part I of the book. An early draft of that part was critically reviewed by Bruce F. Spencer and Willis B. Goldbeck, whose many suggestions added immeasurably to the balance and accuracy of the presentation. Of course, we take full responsibility for any lapses that may remain.

In the preparation of the manuscript, Antonette Doherty and Susan Kelleher handled logistical problems with their usual expertise and dispatch. Janet Marantz edited the contributed papers and in some cases assisted with revisions.

On the series as a whole, Willis B. Goldbeck of the Washington Business Group on Health, and representatives of several member corporations, have served as an important sounding board and source of information and advice. We are extremely grateful for help we have received in the past and welcome input from readers now and in the future.

Boston, November 1978   Richard H. Egdahl

                                                        Diana Chapman Walsh

Contents

I. CONTEXT AND ISSUES   **1**
   Diana Chapman Walsh and Richard H. Egdahl

   1. Industry-Insurer Relationships—A Dynamic Interaction   2

   2. A Spectrum of Financing and Administrative Alternatives   12

   3. Shaving Percentage Points Off Administrative Costs   19

   4. Using Claims Data to Contain Health Care Costs   32

II. PURCHASER PERSPECTIVES: FOUR CORPORATIONS   **53**

   5. American Telephone and Telegraph Company   55
   *Richard W. Stone, Michael J. Gulotta, and Donald P.
   Harrington*

   6. Mobil Oil Corporation   60
   *Robert B. Peters, Jack H. Bleuler, and David H.
   Winkworth*

   7. Deere and Company   65
   Kevin Stokeld

8. Polaroid Corporation   69
   Galt Grant

**III. ADMINISTERING THE BENEFIT: THIRD-PARTY
       VIEWS**   **73**

9. Prudential Insurance Company of America   74
   Lesley L. Ralson

10. Blue Cross-Blue Shield of Greater New York   79
   Steven Sieverts

11. U. S. Administrators   89
   Samuel X. Kaplan

12. United Mine Workers of America Health and Retirement
   Funds   99
   Stephen C. Caulfield

13. United Storeworkers Security Plan   117
   William Michelson and Eleanor J. Tilson

IV. AN ACTION PLAN   **121**
   William J. Bicknell

14. Industry and Insurer Interventions to Control the Costs of
   Health Benefits   122
   William J. Bicknell and Brant Kelch

15. Legal Considerations   163
   John D. Blum

Appendix: Conference Participants Quoted   179

CONTEXT AND ISSUES

Diana Chapman Walsh and Richard H. Egdahl

Industry-Insurer Relationships—A Dynamic Interaction

1

A gradual but accelerating change is taking place in the relationships between carriers of health insurance and their industrial clients. Fiscal arrangements that were nearly universal twenty years ago—conventional insurance coverage with the carrier holding full reserves and administering the plan—have given way to a wide range of alternatives. "Conventional insurance" is no longer the norm.

Health insurance contracts are adapting to a turbulent environment; in concert with their corporate clients, carriers have developed a series of innovations that reflect changing expectations, opportunities, and needs. The innovations, described in chapter 2, aim chiefly at shrinking the segment of the health premium consisting of expenses relating only indirectly, if at all, to claims filed against the plan. These indirect costs include items like state premium tax, risk and profit charges and the investment and cash flow losses to the firm on funds held in reserve by the carrier.

Many firms have worked with their carriers to make some such adjustments in the financing of their health care benefits, and some have made many. A few have by now made most of the refinements possible in the realm of administrative savings, and are approaching the threshold of a qualitatively different kind of innovation—the interventions into the health care delivery system, discussed in chapter 4 and in more detail in chapter 14. Unlike the administrative refinements, which seek to close the gap between the total premium and the amount ultimately paid out in claims, this latter approach attempts to reduce the costs of claims, that is, both the volume and the unit costs of certain medical services.

The possibility that industry, acting independently or in collaboration with private insurance carriers, might implement programs designed to influence the volume of health care services employees demand and use has obvious ramifications for corporate policy and for public policy as well. Emerging as it does as a potential elaboration of an ongoing, evolving relationship between industry and insurer, this possibility is best understood when viewed within that dynamic context. Also, for the many firms still making the transition to the most efficient financing arrangements, there may be valuable practical lessons to be learned from the few that are farthest along. An important caveat, however, is that conditions vary widely from one firm to another—the employee relations of a company comprising mostly office workers versus one that is highly industrialized, the cash flow of a newspaper publisher compared to a swimsuit manufacturer. Before generalizing from a particular company's experiences, one must take these idiosyncracies into account.

The purpose of this monograph is to trace the evolution of the industry-insurer relationship up to the present time, to explore methods by which health care benefits are financed and administered, and to suggest some policy implications that flow from these developments.

Evolving Financing Mechanisms and the Changes They Reflect

As the costs of insuring the benefit have risen, financial and benefits managers have sought ways to assure the highest possible proportion of health services (that is, paid claims) out of the total premium paid the insurer. Responding to this need, and seizing new opportunities uncovered by shifting legal sands, insurers have, over the past fifteen years, developed innovative financing arrangements, such as "minimum premium plans," established in the mid-1960s, and "administrative services only" (ASO) contracts, which began to appear in the early 1970s as an administrative vehicle for a self-funded plan. These modified contracts are described in more detail in chapter 2. The premium is reduced by returning some of the "risk" that the insurer was bearing back to the corporate policyholder, in order to reduce the amount of money the carrier is holding in reserve at any given time and to ease or eliminate entirely the burden of state premium taxes.

The transfer of fiscal responsibility that occurs with these changes, together with steady growth in the sums involved, heightens the industrial manager's awareness of his firm's health care expenses:

> In the past we did little more with data from our carrier than check the addition to make sure the totals were correct. But with the advent of various modified premium arrangements, we as a corporation have assumed more of the risk, and with it, we feel more of the responsibility to monitor the system and control the costs. We find ourselves in the position of any businessman looking at cost centers and profit centers where he's got a lot of money tied up. He wants all the information he can have before making decisions. Because the responsibility to monitor health benefits used to rest totally with the insurance carrier, we have found, as we assume more of these responsibilities, that there's a wealth of information to which we have little access. If this were a normal operations problem with a high priority, we could on any day gather the information needed internally and work it over the next day. Now, when we request information of the insurance carriers, they respond with it to the best of their ability but weeks or even months later and even then, often not exactly as we wanted it. So we're working with the carriers in two spheres—first with the financing of the premium, and secondly with the claims information that we get, so that it will be more timely and more useful to us as we plan for the future.
>
> John L. Bauer, Jr.*

A subtly shifting mandate such as Bauer describes is an important but somewhat subjective influence. A more concrete reason for the corporation to begin looking beyond the administrative balance sheet to the health care system itself is the growing realization, among firms that have adopted streamlined funding schemes, that they may already have seen whatever savings they can anticipate. And yet costs continue to rise. Administrative refinements designed to squeeze the "fat" out of the insurance contract bring the firm quite soon to a plateau of cost savings, above which it is difficult to progress without confronting the reality, encapsulated by Jacob J. Spies for the first volume of this series:

> The insurance premium, really, is a function of health care costs, and not the other way around. As we talk about these kinds of negotiations with insurance companies, we have to remember that there are deeper problems that we should be getting through to.

Few deny the importance of Spies's point. The differences arise over just how far to push the negotiations on administrative savings—where, exactly is the plateau? These differences reflect, in turn, divided opinion as to the most effective means of reaching that optimal level of savings as quickly as possible. The most radical departure from a conventionally insured approach is represented by self-insurance, that is, self-funding of the benefit and self-administration of the claims. But, as detailed in chapter 3, there are conflicting views of the administrative money to be saved through these mechanisms. Beyond administrative savings, however, the trend toward self-insurance of

*See appendix for affiliations of quoted conference participants.

health benefits—if indeed it is a trend—is attracting attention as a possible influence on the overall costs of medical care in America. There are two related reasons for this general public policy interest.

Self-Insurance as an Issue of Public Policy

Public policy interest in self-insurance derives first from impending decisions about national health insurance, which must include judgments about where the private health insurance industry will fit into a national plan.

> The relationships between the large employers and their health insurance carriers have tremendous implications for national health insurance. It is not immediately clear how a national plan should be managed. Many worry that the federal government can't do it. It doesn't look like the states can or will do it; nor can the providers do it alone, nor the Blues. No one has the answer, specifically. Difficult as it may be for some to accept, our health system will probably never be truly centralized. The implications of what services industry really wants from insurers are very, very important for what's being discussed in Washington right now. In this sense, industry (management and labor) has the same needs as government in its role as a major purchaser of insurance: good data; speedy, equitable claims processing; assistance in monitoring provider performance; a benefit package designed to produce the best possible health outcomes for the most reasonable cost. The extent to which industry can reorder its priorities and obtain such services from the carriers will have a major impact on the extent of future government regulation in health.
>
> Willis B. Goldbeck

The prospect of some form of national health insurance plan certainly clouds the carriers' crystal ball, but also that of corporate financial and risk managers who wonder whether it is worth their time and effort to restructure the financing of the private health benefit plan that may shortly be discontinued or profoundly altered. But, then again it may not and meanwhile the costs are high. These deliberations reflect on the carriers' role.

If it is true that self-insurance is growing in popularity among the nation's large employers, does this mean that some of the carriers' most sophisticated clients are discovering that they can do a more efficient and effective job of managing the health benefit by either bringing the administration in-house or contracting with a noninsurance firm that specializes in administration only? Critics of the insurance industry would say yes, that self-insurance is prima facie evidence that the carriers are insufficiently flexible to meet the changing needs of their large corporate policyholders. But is it fair to draw this conclusion without asking what kinds of innovation their corporate clients have demanded and are now demanding? The insurance industry spokesmen quoted in the first box suggest that the demand for cost containment is a relatively recent phenomenon, which even now seems out of step with the

ARE THE CARRIERS PUSHING . . .

Bruce F. Spencer: An essential question is what have corporate health insurance policyholders been asking their carriers for in the way of cost control.

Michael P. McDonald: Speaking for Blue Cross, I can say that clients are interested in general but that very few have actually asked for special programs. We volunteer much more than clients ask for—which is not necessarily to say that we volunteer enough—but we often get the message: "Do all these things to intervene and to restrain the rates of increase, but don't get my employees shaken up when they have a claim."

Joseph W. Mullen, Jr.: In the past three to five years, we at Metropolitan Life have been finding keen interest among our large accounts for cost containment programs. It used to be that the corporations only wanted financial accounting information; now more and more want utilization data.

Lesley L. Ralson: I have some trouble with the implication that the insurance industry has had to be dragged kicking and screaming into the twentieth century. Over a number of years the Prudential has developed various ways to restructure the benefit so as to contain costs, but they didn't sell. We developed the capacity to produce utilization data some ten years ago, but very few customers have used it. One of our clients has been paying a person for nine years to work on cost containment, but that's the exception. Overall, we are now seeing greatly increased interest in cost control, but it's still less than we'd like to see.

Gordon W. Thomas: Certainly, major clients of the Hancock are interested in cost control. But our medium-sized to smaller clients, by and large, are still focusing on premiums or on the savings in the so-called retention dollar, the taxes, the reserves, and cash flow implications. I am not sure that cost control is in appropriately sharp focus for any but the very large accounts. It is the rare account that is looking beyond the administrative costs to the delivery system itself.

. . . OR BEING PUSHED?

John L. Brown: As of now, I have no quarrel with the relationship between Genesco and our insurance carriers; our sense of urgency about costs has increased and the carriers have responded. About two years ago we approached our home office carrier—Blue Cross-Blue Shield—for assistance in controlling some abuse we had discovered through our own data collection effort and at first found them very reluctant. It appeared that we were the first employer who had come forward with this type of request. However, once we got started into our program, the carrier became very supportive, indeed welcomed the chance to take part. Now we are extending our programs into other parts of the country, and are finding enthusiasm and cooperation.

Timothy B. Sullivan: I find it interesting that in Mr. Brown's success story, Genesco did the data analysis themselves. When I asked my carrier—John Hancock—for Balfour's data, the agent asked what I wanted to do with it and what kinds of questions I had. I thought that should have fallen within the carrier's technical assistance services—but I came up with five or six examples of the kinds of things I'd like to know about, and in response I received two and a half inches of computer print-out. Evidently, it is up to me to have that analyzed, but I think the carrier should do that analysis.

Gordon W. Thomas: I'm with the Hancock and I agree with you 100 percent. We will analyze that data for you. We will help you identify utilization patterns, frequency of use, the hot spots that are causing you problems.

Sullivan: Those are the questions I asked and I got this two and a half inches back.

Thomas: We'll do this analysis for any client that asks.

Richard H. Egdahl: And for all the clients that do not ask?

Thomas: No, because we would have to assess the costs against all employers; many would find them excessive.

William J. Bicknell: But is there not an obligation on the part of the insurer to try to create some interest and awareness? The health insurance business is intimately involved with the health care delivery system, while the corporate policyholder has but a very peripheral involvement. It seems to me that educating policyholders might be a very worthwhile effort on the part of some of the carriers.

desires of the ultimate consumers—employees:

> We have to remember that an employer's purchase of health care
> coverage is entirely different from his purchase of, say, paper
> towels. Employers think of the dollars that they are spending,
> whether through self-insurance, a commercial carrier, or a Blues
> plan, as their dollars, while employees view them as their dollars
> that have been bargained for either directly or by proxy, and would
> be going into direct wages if they were not going into health insur-
> ance. The average employee has strong feelings about what he or she
> wants from health care and health insurance, and these complicate
> the employer's problem.
>
> Steven Sieverts

The perspectives of the health insurance purchasers, represented in the second box, suggest that corporate policyholders are not necessarily blaming the insurance industry for past omissions, but some are now looking for greater innovation. The carriers assert that they have served their clients well, and ask whether there is some social obligation on their industry to try to create a demand for more rigorous cost containment than the public seems ready to accept. If so, they ask, from whence does the mandate come? These questions cannot be dismissed lightly.

One important focus of policy interest, then, is what lessons—if any—may be inferred from self-insurance for the prospective place of the private carriers in a national health insurance program? Some role for them is now virtually as-sured, whatever the specifics of the plan finally enacted. But complex issues remain to be resolved before there can be a plan. The particulars of the role to be reserved for the private carriers—both the commercial firms and Blue Cross-Blue Shield—and how the government will regulate them are far from resolved.

The second source of general interest in the self-insurance experience is a particular lesson it is thought by some to harbor. The assertion is sometimes made that when a corporation or union elects to fund or administer its own health benefits it has stronger incentives and better information to make the transition from a passive payer for health care to an aggressive purchaser, willing and able to intervene in the health system and challenge unreasonable costs. Bicknell and Kelch espouse "system intervention" in chapter 14 of this volume. Theirs is an advocacy position, implying that whether or not firms actually are gravitating toward self-insurance, they should be if they and the nation are to contain rising health care costs.

A similar view of self-insurance permeated a widely quoted 1976 report of the President's Council on Wage and Price Stability.[1] The report focused on the rising costs of health care and the potential role of the private sector in bringing them under control. Quoting data collected by the Washington Business Group on Health and describing the activities of Goodyear Tire and Rubber Company, the report suggested that undertaking self-insurance draws a corporation into the health planning process:

> Goodyear also pays its medical bills directly, rather than buying health care
> insurance (except for prescription drug benefits). Aside from the adminis-

trative savings that flow from this arrangement, it probably carries a certain psychological impact: direct participation in planning the health care system would seem to be a legitimate role for an organization that actually pays the bills generated by that system. "Self-insurance" also gives Goodyear direct and immediate access to claims data, which can be helpful in the planning process, as well as sole responsibility for individual claims review. Goodyear's approach, then, is holistic in a double sense. First, the company is involved in every aspect of controlling costs—the costs of benefits administration, of unwarranted individual claims, of system-wide patterns of inappropriate utilization and of building health care facilities. Second, Goodyear focuses on the system, not particular practitioners, hospitals or medical procedures. The company's emphasis is on altering general patterns of health care delivery rather than reducing individual claims that may not be fully warranted. . . . Claims monitoring and reporting also provide needed information for intelligent and credible participation in planning.[2]

Elsewhere, the report posited a relationship between self-insurance and an inclination to innovate in the realm of reimbursement of physicians and hospitals:

Self-insurance is a misnomer which actually means that the benefit plan does not pay premiums to an insurance company for health coverage, but pays providers directly. This can save administrative costs, taxes—which an insurance company must pay but a benefit plan need not—and other relatively small costs. It also gives benefit plan administrators direct control of health care provider reimbursement and thus puts administrators in position to work with providers on controlling costs.[3]

Two of the cases touched upon in the council's examination of provider reimbursement are updated and expanded in part III of this volume: the United Storeworkers Union Security Plan and the United Mine Workers of America Health and Retirement Funds.

Another indirect advantage the council saw flowing from self-insurance arises in the context of the Storeworkers' program of providing coverage for a second surgical opinion for beneficiaries contemplating elective surgery:

The method of enforcing pre-surgical review is important too. Self-insurance . . . gives employee benefit administrators timely access to information on members scheduled for surgery. About 25 percent of those Storeworkers Fund members who call the second opinion intake workers do so only after being reminded of the program when they call the Fund's Hospitalization Department.[4]

The council suspended its enthusiasm for self-insurance just long enough to give passing mention to opposing viewpoints, but returned quickly to endorse self-insurance for companies really desiring to become actively engaged in containing costs:

On the other hand, insurance companies and their larger clients have developed means of reducing some of these *extra* [administrative and tax] costs substantially. And for many clients, smaller ones especially, health insurance itself performs vital functions: risk pooling, prospective budgeting of benefit costs, and expert handling of health care claims. For small and large clients alike, the start-up costs and organizational demands of "self-insurance" are substantial. These demands are particularly onerous for an employer that would prefer not to get involved in employee health care—an employer that prefers to have an insurance company act as buffer between itself and its employees. However, this is precisely the most important advantage of "self-insurance" to Goodyear—direct company involvement.[5]

Goodyear is often cited as a firm that has exhibited unusual commitment to the goal of containing health care costs without compromising quality. Commitment is a central tenet in the "systems intervention" case for self-insurance, which builds on assumptions about concentration of power, the ability or inclination to act, and how these factors may relate to being self-insured. Here, as elsewhere, opinion is sharply divided. Some argue, with the Council on Wage and Price Stability and with Kevin Stokeld of Deere and Company in chapter 7, that being self-insured stiffens the spine, enhances the firm's expertise, and unleashes its creativity. Others suspect that the effects of mere financing arrangements cannot be so fundamental. They point to corporations like Ford Motor Company and General Motors where the "buffer" of an insurance carrier has not seemed to diminish the firm's commitment, creativity, and leadership in pursuit of health care cost containment. They very much doubt that self-insurance alone can appreciably alter the incentives facing industry:

> Self-insurance makes good sense in certain situations. But I do not believe that simply because the benefits manager for John Deere or any other company suddenly has claims clerks working for him, that he will have more power or more incentive to do something about health care delivery. Industrial executives have the power now, if they want to act. The executives of one corporation I recently visited in a town where there is a single medical center hold sixteen seats on that hospital's board of directors. That firm does not need to hire claims clerks in order to have leverage in that medical community. I hope we do not rush into self-insurance as a panacea; I think it is really a nitty administrative savings issue—the kind of issue that cost accountants will ultimately decide.
>
> Thomas O. Pyle

Even confirmed advocates of self-insurance agree that it is no panacea, that it serves only as a means to an end. It may provide a vehicle for beginning to influence the costs of claims, and specifically the utilization of health care services. To do so requires information on patterns of practice and patterns of use. The struggle over data brings the industry-insurer relationship beyond the circumscribed arena of internal business policy and into the public realm. To the administrator of health benefits fall essential choices about what information to collect, how, and why. These color subsequent determinations of how claims are to be adjudicated and paid, on what grounds they may be challenged, and who will set the ground rules. Embedded in the answers are potential implications for the future of the health insurance industry, and more generally for the practice patterns of all providers of health care and the shape of the future delivery system.

Industry has a distinct perspective on these questions and a large stake in the outcome. As the major purchaser of private health insurance for employees and their dependents, industry has long been in a dynamic interaction with the insurance carriers. This puts industry in a unique position to help shape future policy.

Whoever administers the benefit—whether insurance carrier, claims administrator, health and welfare fund administrators, or the firm itself—will face the problem of how to collect data, how much to invest in its acquisition and processing, how to display and interpret it, with whom to share it, and, most important, how to use it to contain costs without compromising quality. Thus the initial question—when, why, and how should a company consider the option of self-insuring its employee health benefit plan?—requires a careful analysis.

A Spectrum of Financing and Administrative Alternatives

The funding alternatives available for an employee health care plan range from conventional insurance with the carrier or service plan bearing the risk, holding full reserves, and administering the claims, to an entirely uninsured or self-insured plan, where the employer or union assumes all these functions. Between the two poles lies a wide spectrum of possibilities and hybrids, most developed within the past fifteen years.

The funding choice fixes the administrative mechanism and often takes account not only of direct fiscal constraints on the firm or health and welfare fund, but also of indirect factors such as corporate or union philosophy, the preferences, characteristics, and geographic distribution of employees, the design and scope of the benefit package, and so on. For a large firm, consequently, the decision may cut across the domains of the financial department, the personnel and/or industrial relations departments, and, to a lesser but growing extent, the medical department as well.

> *I find real differences in the orientations of different functional
> units within a firm—personnel, employee relations, insurance
> manager, or financial officer. They have disparate viewpoints here,
> viewing fringe benefits from different perspectives, and very differ-
> ent perceptions of the need to contain health costs. The level of
> interest you find depends to a great extent on whom you are dealing
> with.*
>
> Bernard T. Hurley, Jr.

Balancing these diverse and sometimes conflicting orientations, while
keeping sight of obligations to employees, stockholders, providers of health
care, and the wider community, complicates the task not only of the carrier,
broker, or consultant, as Hurley implies, but also of individuals within the firm
with pieces of the responsibility for the decision.

Elements of the consideration are treated later in this volume, especially
in chapter 14 by Bicknell and Kelch, which includes a table summarizing the
major funding alternatives and the salient differences among them. For comprehensive discussions of historical antecedents, legal complexities, fiscal sub-
tleties, and administrative implications of various funding options, the *Employee Benefit Plan Review Research Reports*[6] are an excellent source, as is
Bruce Spencer's recently updated book.[7] Spencer's *Employee Benefit Plan
Review*[8] and another trade publication, *Business Insurance*[9], frequently feature
short articles describing the experiences of various employee health benefit
programs and issues aired at conferences, including some the publishers themselves have organized. The American Management Association and the Risk
and Insurance Management Society, Inc. also run frequent conferences and
training sessions for professional managers of employee benefits. The Conference Board[10] does so too—although somewhat less often.

A standard health insurance text would be of value to the uninitiate for a
systematic approach to basic definitions and concepts.[11] The publications of
the Health Insurance Institute, including its annual source books, serve similar
uses.[12]

The first volume in the Industry and Health Care series briefly sketches
the background of the health insurance industry, describes some causes and
effects of rising costs, and surveys approaches to cost containment currently in
vogue. That discussion concludes:

> Cost containment activities are being tried by industry in a variety of forms
> and settings and under various auspices. Considerable ingenuity is manifest
> in many of these efforts and some appear promising, although few have
> produced irrefutable evidence of effectiveness. Little is known about over-
> lapping effects the various strategies may have nor about their possible
> unintended side effects both within the health system and beyond. For
> example, the gains in system-wide efficiency of closing down a community
> hospital may be lost in unemployment. Most of the cost containment
> strategies developed to date have ardent supporters and equally convinced
> detractors. And most appear either to require a major commitment of time
> and energy, which will have to be sustained over a period of years before
> results can reasonably be expected, or else to promise a quick but relatively
> minor payoff. The challenge will be to sort through these various pos-

sibilities, identify the ones that are best suited to local circumstances, and arrive at a comprehensive and well thought out approach that makes the most sense for the particular firm or union, for its employees or rank and file, and for the broader community of which it is a member.[13]

An annotated bibliography accompanying that volume cites additional sources of information bearing on industry's role as payer for health care.

Rather than duplicate material available elsewhere, then, the purpose of this section is to establish as concisely as possible a frame of reference and common vocabulary for the remainder of the volume.

Alternatives Evolve

Experience rating opened the door for the innovations culminating in self-insurance by diminishing the carrier's assumption of risk. In chapter 9 Ralson of the Prudential makes this connection and observes that experience rating was "the commercial insurance industry's first major innovation in the employee benefits field." Blue Cross plans originally used community-rating systems whereby a single rate was set for all potential individual and group members in an area, generally without reference to actuarial projections of differences in risk according to age, sex, occupation, and status of health. Beginning in the 1940s and 1950s, and in some places continuing to the present, commercial carriers were able to outcompete the Blues by offering an employed group an experience rate based on its actual and projected experience, usually entailing a substantially lower premium.

Another practical impact of experience rating was the effect it began to have on the negotiations between financial officers of large firms and their insurance carriers. Large accounts with stable work forces experienced relatively minor fluctuations in the volume of claims, and the annual increase in the experience-rated premium was easily predicted by applying a standard medical care inflation factor to the previous year's premium. This straightforward relationship brought home the fact that the insurance carrier was relieving the firm of little risk, except perhaps to protect one-year cash flow. In effect, the beneficiary groups covered by large corporations had grown to such a size as to render irrelevant the essential function of insurance, that is, reducing risk by pooling independent exposures. A logical next step was to begin questioning insurers' reserve requirements, about which the carriers had been rather vague up through the 1960s.[14]

The "turning point" in this process, according to the *Employee Benefit Plan Review Research Reports,* came at a 1964 meeting of the American Management Association:

> Since that time, benefits managers and financial officers of corporations have become increasingly aware of the financial aspects of health care coverage. In turn, many insurance companies and service plans have responded with improved claims service, more complete financial reporting and a closer evaluation of the true reserve requirements.[15]

A focus of attention at the 1964 meeting was the prototype minimum premium plan—"Cat-Met," which the Metropolitan Life Insurance Company had previously developed with Caterpillar Tractor. From then on, despite legal and regulatory perturbations well into the 1970s, successive generations of minimum premium arrangements evolved and flourished, and carriers other than Metropolitan created their own variations on the minimum premium theme. Among these was the Equitable Life Assurance Society, which altered the minimum premium concept in 1970 by writing a contract with the 3-M Company in St. Paul, Minnesota, stipulating that 3-M would bear the risk and the Equitable would provide administrative services only. ASO subsequently emerged as a common method of administering a self-funded benefit plan.

Two congressional initiatives round out the historical background. The Tax Reform Act of 1969 included, as one of many provisions, changes in section 501(c)(9) of the Internal Revenue Code, enabling firms to accumulate interest-bearing reserves in a tax-exempt vehicle that is characterized as the purest form of self-funded arrangements, a 501(c)(9) trust.[16] Five years later, Congress enacted the pension reform act (ERISA), which includes, in section 514(b), an apparent preemption of state regulation of uninsured benefit plans. Preemption is still the subject of much legal debate, as reported by Blum in chapter 15, but ERISA does insulate self-funded plans from many of the burdens of state regulation.

Naturally, these innovations developed first in the context of the very large accounts whose beneficiary groups were large enough that aggregate risks were small, and who were best equipped to absorb some fluctuations in cash flow. Gradually, though, some of the principles have filtered down to smaller and smaller firms—and some observers predict that this trend may continue.[17]

Choosing Among Alternatives

In chapter 14, Bicknell and Kelch trace the thought sequence involved in choosing among funding mechanisms. The choice requires isolating and contrasting the three major elements of insurance-related costs: reserve requirements and the method for crediting earnings on reserves; risk charges and retentions; and taxes. These three elements, sometimes factored out differently, are used to weigh the relative merits and administrative costs of various funding options. Their implications are treated in some detail by Bicknell and Kelch; the controversy they engender is the subject of chapter 3.

Although there are many combinations and permutations, the major options available can be grouped in five broad categories, along a spectrum from greatest insurance company involvement to least:

(1) *Conventional full insurance.* The carrier collects a premium (usually experience-rated), underwrites the risk of unexpected fluctuations in claims, and provides administrative services including such things as enrolling employees, filling out government forms, producing summary

plan descriptions and other communication vehicles, providing actuarial and legal services, and related activities.

The premium includes an actuarily determined amount earmarked for claim payments, plus a *retention* to cover the insurance company's cost of doing business. A useful way to think about the alternative funding arrangements is to consider them as devices to reduce the numerical difference—"the gap"—between the premium and the amount the carrier ultimately pays out in claims.[18] This gap consists of: state premium *taxes* (typically about 2 percent of the premium); *administrative* charges; *risk* charges (chiefly to protect the carrier should the contract be terminated with insufficient reserves to pay incurred claims); brokers' commissions; and so on. Also in the premium is an allowance for *reserves* to protect against an abnormally high volume of claims at any time during the course of the contract. State insurance departments require that carriers hold a certain level of reserves, the actual amount varying by state and by type of plan. In conventional health insurance it tends to run at about 20 percent of paid claims per year, and sometimes somewhat higher.

Even under a fully insured plan, special arrangements can be negotiated with the carrier to compensate the policyholder for his loss of earnings on reserves, for example, a two- or three-month lag before the first payment comes due, interim accounting methods to adjust the reserve level midway through the policy year, retrospective arrangements obligating the employer to make up any deficit in the account should reserves prove to be insufficient, use of reserves as compensating balances on bank accounts or acceptance of securities in lieu of cash payments. However, it is usually the case that reserve modifications are undertaken in combination with an alternative to fully-insured coverage, doubtless because employers who know to inquire about the former are also likely to opt for the latter.

(2) **Minimum premium plan.** Developed principally to reduce state premium taxes, which it does in most but not all states, this arrangement retains for the carrier essentially the same role as in a conventionally insured plan, performing the full complement of underwriting, claims processing, and administrative services. There is a contract, which can be important for collective bargaining purposes, and the carrier issues a master group insurance policy to the employer and certificates of insurance to employees.

The essential difference appears in an amendment to the contract, where the carrier and the policyholder each agree to assume a specified share of the claims liability. Typically, the policyholder's "maximum dollar limit" above which the insurer will pay is set as a percentage (often 90 percent) of "expected claims," that is the level of claims anticipated, on the basis of previous years' experience. The expected level is set high so that the employer usually carries the full responsibility. In one type of minimum premium plan, the policyholder pays to this ceiling each month; in another he pays all the claims throughout the contract year until he reaches an annual maximum. The former is normally preferred by the policyholder for its obvious cash flow advantages.

The employer's liability for paying the bulk of claims accounts for the minimal premium. It needs to cover only the tax, risk, and profit charges associated with the carrier's share of the liability, a small fraction of the base on which these charges would otherwise be calculated. The carrier does establish reserves for the full risk of the account, since he bears ultimate responsibility should the policyholder go out of business.[19]

(3) *Self-funding with an administrative services only (ASO) contract.* ASO is not a financing mechanism per se, but a device for administering a self-funded plan. It involves no assumption of risk by a third-party insurer, and reserves are established independently by the employer or through a 501(c)(9) trust. The plan is "self-insured," or, to be more precise, "self-funded," since insurance is absent. Few states currently tax uninsured health benefit plans, and for now at least, state regulation of such plans appears to be largely preempted by ERISA (see chapter 15 by Blum). Contracts do not have to be filed with the state insurance commissioners, which can give a large multi-state employer, with different coverages in different states, considerably more flexibility in the design (and redesign) of his benefit plan.[20] Review of claims, data collection, plan design, and other administrative duties are contracted out to a third-party, often an insurance carrier or a contract administrator, like U.S. Administrators, described in chapters 4 and 11.

(4) *Stop-loss coverage.* Normally purchased from a carrier or contract administrator in conjunction with claims administration, stop-loss coverage protects the otherwise self-insured policyholder against excessive claims, either on an aggregate basis or in an individual case. Premiums are minimized under this plan, along with premium taxes and reserves. But stop-loss coverage can be expensive.

(5) *Self-funding and self-administration.* This is the other extreme of the spectrum from conventional coverage. With or without a 501(c)(9) trust, the employer or multi-employer trust takes on all the administrative functions associated with the health benefit.

Deere and Company, described in chapter 7, has elected self-administration. Kevin Stokeld of Deere is a "true believer" and the observation he makes merits further attention:

> It makes so much sense for many large corporations that I am really surprised self-insurance isn't more prevalent.
>
> Kevin Stokeld

Stokeld's comment raises the question of how widespread self-funding and self-administration really is. Little hard evidence is available with which to fashion a definitive response. The Washington Business Group on Health did a quick survey in December 1975 and reported to the Council on Wage and Price Stability:

> Goldbeck . . . found that of 93 companies providing insurance for medical benefits, 8 were fully self-insured and 19 partially self-insured. Half of these

companies began self-insuring for medical benefits within the past five years. Perhaps more significant is the trend: an additional 18 firms expect to switch to self-insurance in the future.[21]

Recently, the Office of Policy, Planning, and Research of the Department of Health, Education, and Welfare's Health Care Financing Administration has contracted with Westat, Inc., to conduct a national survey of independent prepaid and self-insured health plans. A "screener questionnaire" was mailed in August 1978, and the project will not be completed for about a year, whereupon it will produce a central repository for information on uninsured health plans. Meanwhile, data is sketchy but it is safe to say, as Spencer does in his book, that there is a discernible movement, even among smaller companies, away from conventional funding arrangements where the carrier held full reserves: "By the mid-1970s, some companies with just a few employees had changed their methods of financing health care benefits—often from fully insured plans to plans that were substantially noninsured, but with some type of stop-loss arrangement in the event of an unusual claim."[22] He also predicts that this motion will accelerate: "The interest in the financing of group benefits will continue and will affect many of those who have, up to this point, been primarily involved with fully insured plans."[23] To what extent this constitutes a trend away from the private carriers may at present be a policy issue that cannot be fully solved. In any event, it seems clear that both industry and insurer are feeling mounting pressure to implement financing options that reduce as far as possible the insurance-related costs of providing the employee health benefit.

Shaving Percentage Points Off Administrative Costs

3

How much money should a firm or health and welfare fund expect to save by moving away from full insurance? This sounds like a straightforward question that ought to yield to a fairly objective answer, based on a range of experiences. Instead, the answer seems strangely elusive and tangled in individual opinion. One problem is time and the press of expanding responsibilities—few managers have adequate time to spend in sharing business experiences and knowledge with others in analogous circumstances. Another is the complexity of the question and the number of variables involved. Each firm is different and the only safe way to estimate the potential cost savings is to dissect them into component parts and talk in terms of ranges, with a margin for error. But this approach introduces other errors, since the component parts are in some ways inseparable. Money saved in one sphere may well reappear, whether recognized or not, as money lost in another.

The two components of the premium—the monies allocated for administration and those dedicated to paying claims—are inseparable. Trade-offs make it impossible to look at one in isolation and then move on to the other. I would especially caution against overlooking the dimensions to administration that are much neglected at the moment: quality assurance, utilization review, data evaluation, consumer education, and things of that kind. Eventually, we ought to look at the indirect costs of illness that do not show up as medical care costs, but as costs to society and to employers—absenteeism, loss of productivity, disability, rehabilitation, welfare dependency, and a whole array of other dimensions that are the effects of illness. It is important—however difficult—to consider all the costs.

Geoffrey V. Heller

Bearing in mind that there are contaminations across categories of cost, it is still worthwhile to try to take them apart and examine them one by one.

State Premium Taxes and the Issue of Societal Subsidy

Given that state premium taxes can usually be reduced or eliminated by taking the relatively short step from conventional insurance to a minimum premium plan, is there any reason for a firm to be paying this tax? The answer depends upon the perspective. For some firms state premium taxes have probably been a decisive factor in their move away from conventional insurance, for the simple reason that for some accounts, with the retention already fairly well reduced to a minimum, taxes represented a highly visible component of the carrier's remaining retention, that could be disposed of summarily:

In very simplistic terms there are really only three identifiable parts of the financing package: Claims, reserves, and retention. For a large company, premium taxes constitute 40–50 percent of the retention. In one very simple stroke the benefits manager can eliminate up to half the retention and that's what makes self-insurance look so attractive.

James H. Brennan, Jr.

Complicating the issues, particularly for multi-state employers, is the fact that some states, such as Connecticut and Idaho, do levy a tax on uninsured employee health benefits, which is tantamount to a premium tax although no premium is actually involved. As this volume went to press, the Connecticut law was in court. Depending on the resolution of this case, other states might follow suit or find other ways of recovering the revenues they lose as more and more firms adopt the arrangements that shelter them from state premium taxes:

Sure, there are ways to avoid taxes, but doesn't that just extend the question? If everybody pursues that end, then finally the state

misses the revenue and raises it through some other source. Since it is easier to tax corporations and businesses and since the state legislature recognizes these premium taxes were coming from businesses, they will no doubt raise the corporate tax. In the long run, you may have transferred the burden in a different form to different individual companies, but not in the aggregate, reduced it. The state needs the revenue and will eventually find a way to get it.
                                                          Michael P. McDonald

In response to McDonald's prediction, one can argue that the relative lack of movement in this direction over the past fifteen years would seem to discredit it as a burgeoning trend. Related to the question of state taxes are three important issues, none with simple answers, but all warranting attention. First is the tax policy itself and the undesired, unforeseen, even still largely unrecognized effect it may be having on a segment of the economy:

Here is another example of tax policy distorting behavior in our economy. Obviously, a profit-center manager with a time horizon of about twelve months would really want to get rid of the 2 percent. If you could step away from that distortion, it would be recognized as an artifact of the tax law which could be changed next year to suddenly make it very disadvantageous to self-insure.
                                                          Thomas O. Pyle

Second, one can ask to what uses those taxes are being put, how well they are serving the public interest, and whether the government should penalize a firm that is contributing to the public good by providing health insurance.

I would raise a different question about premium taxes. With the interest in reducing taxes that we saw in California in the Proposition 13 referendum, maybe we should consider doing away with all state insurance departments and the taxes along with them. The number of them that serve a useful function for an employee health benefits plan probably could be counted on the fingers of one hand.
                                                          Bruce F. Spencer

Third, the issue of taxes—society's explicit mechanism for financing public services and, in effect, redistributing wealth—points to similar questions of implicit or hidden cross-subsidies that may be taking place in the health insurance relationship. They may be offsetting the effect of the explicit tax policy, or largely reinforcing it, probably some combination; to some extent they may have developed in reaction to it. But whatever their origins and effects, they belong on the public agenda. One congressional staff member raised these issues:

I have two questions. First, would carriers that offer more than one line of insurance tend to make up any losses in health in a given year by simply increasing the cost to the corporation in other lines? My other question is related. From the standpoint of society, should we worry that the costs to smaller companies or even larger ones

that cannot or will not self-insure are going to go up as big com-
panies pull out and do self-insure? Could the aggregate costs to
society for health insurance end up increasing as a result of, let us
say, government encouragement of self-insurance?

Harvey Pies

Somewhat related to these two questions raised by Pies is a third—
whether there is competition in the insurance industry and if so, what are the
essential differences, from the standpoint of society, between Blue Cross-Blue
Shield on the one hand and the commercial carriers on the other? The distinction
traditionally drawn between the Blues and the commercial carriers has rested on
historical developments touched on in the first volume of this series. As nonprofit entities, the Blues have achieved an aura of "community service" in return
for which, in most states, they pay no premium tax. In lieu of that tax, however,
the Blues subsidize nongroup coverage by maintaining open enrollment for
individuals throughout the year:

Blue Cross is tax-exempt in part because one-fourth to one-third of
our total membership consists of small groups and individual
policies: people who for all practical purposes are out of the market
for commercial health insurance. Most plans have year-round open
enrollment for individual subscribers, a category where we know
we are going to lose money every year. We provide supplementary
coverage for Medicare beneficiaries, where we know in advance
that we are going to be paying out more than a dollar for every
dollar we take in. We are proud of this; it is a price we pay for
important privileges from state government and the marketplace.
Mr. Pies is posing a very serious question when he asks whether the
push of major industry to save dollars on retention could become
so strong as to jeopardize this community role of Blue Cross-Blue
Shield. Blue Cross could not continue this role without a large
population base, and it's my firm conviction that employers have a
societal responsibility here that goes beyond their immediate em-
ployees.

Steven Sieverts

Some policyholders may not share the sense of mission Sieverts ex-
presses. Instead they may view the Blues' community subsidy as a hidden tax,
offering little or nothing in return. But there are compensations, as the AT&T
discussion in chapter 5 points out, in particular the hospital discounts that the
Blues pass on to their members. As a closely regulated utility with an enormous
employee population and unique financial leverage, AT&T may be especially
mindful of the ripple effect its internal decisions about health care benefits
could have on the wider health care delivery system. However, most of the
corporations large enough to consider self-funding and self-administering a
health benefit are conscious of the secondary effects that their decisions could
have:

The kind of corporation that might self-insure would tend to be
visible, to say the least. They are major entities in their political

*environments. One program that I've been involved with has vol-
untarily paid premium taxes on a self-insured program, because we
felt it would be a political error to attempt to avoid them. Any
program on the part of large corporations that could be viewed as
avoiding taxes might run into some political problems.*

Thomas O. Pyle

By paying full hospital charges, the commercial carriers on behalf of their
corporate policyholders are, in effect, picking up a share of the bad debt in
hospital budgets that the government will not pay—another subtle subsidy.
Pies's question is probing whether they remain competitive by using health
insurance as a loss leader in a multiple-line business. Direct cross-subsidies are
illegal, according to representatives of the industry, who nevertheless seem to
imply that the law may leave room for subtler kinds of shifting:

*Multiple line companies would encounter legal problems if after
the fact they attempted to divert a loss from health over to product
liability or Workers' Compensation. However, some lines are
traditionally more profitable than others, and health insurance is
one of the least. So before the fact, in rate making and dividends,
carriers can, in an anticipatory way, in a sense, subsidize. For
instance, many companies writing health and life will to the extent
legally possible not write health without life, because life tends to
be more predictable than health. But insurers may not use
hindsight to say that they are going to recoup the money this year
on product liability that they are losing on health.*

Robert F. Froehlke

*John Hancock's accounting practices are probably illustrative of
carriers in the life and health business, though not of casualty
lines, which we don't write. We allocate our charges on an equitable basis to all classes of business that we write; we do not necessarily expect one class of business to support the overhead for other
classes. If we lose money on our group health line, then the group
health line takes the loss and we expect to recover that loss from
the group health line in future years. I think it is as simple as that. I
do not think we expect that our individual business will subsidize
our group business one bit.*

Gordon W. Thomas

Another subtle factor that is in some ways analogous to cross-subsidization
across lines of business is in the matter of corporate borrowing, discussed in
the *Employee Benefit Plan Review Research Reports:*

Corporate borrowing is important in many industries, and insurers are a
prime source of funds. Even though a good argument for self-insurance might
be made, the senior executive of a corporation may be reluctant to cut a line of
credit. For this reason, plans that retain some insurance company involvement are usually preferable. However . . . insurance companies [are changing]
their tunes regarding group health insurance. Few insurers are willing to
haggle over the size of a rate increase any more; health care losses are just too

great. This new-found independence appears to be influencing the corporate borrowing considerations as well; some carriers are quite willing to make loans, even in the period of "tight money," or show no inclination to relate the loan to the employer's group coverage.[24]

As with financial accounting that mixes separate lines of business, the use of corporate lending as a lever in the insurance marketplace is circumscribed legally. But, again, there may be subtler effects that are entirely legal but that distort the incentives in the health care system.

One other tacit subsidy that self-insurance brings into sharp relief is the somewhat ambiguous question of the impact the smaller firms may feel as a result of larger firms' efforts to contain their own health care costs. On one hand there is little doubt, in answer to Pies's second question, that as the larger firms tighten their financing arrangements, the carriers will recover some of their losses from smaller accounts:

> *The nature of experience rating is that as a certain risk pool does better, there is a tendency for others to do worse. So it is likely that as we get more competitive on the larger risk, the smaller risk may pick up more costs.*
>
> Robert F. Froehlke

On the other hand, it can be argued that the large accounts can lead the way to improvements that will eventually save money for all:

> *I have a different view of the subsidization of the smaller company by the larger. I think any progress that can be made by intervention in the health delivery system will have a favorable impact on health care costs overall. To the extent that large corporations lead in that struggle and achieve some results, the impact will be felt all the way down the line, even by very small employers.*
>
> John Hickey

> *The impact will depend on the kind of intervention you are talking about. Many interventions I have heard discussed focus somewhat narrowly; an HMO that may serve only a large company, for example.*
>
> Harvey Pies

> *Perhaps. But if companies with a large concentration of employees find they have more potential for containing costs through an HMO than through other direct interventions, then smaller employers in those same areas will still benefit from those activities. I do not believe that experience rating means that reducing the cost of the large employer necessarily would elevate the costs of the smaller employers. I think it could go in the same direction.*
>
> John Hickey

The diversity of opinion demonstrates that the question of paying state premium taxes is not nearly as simple as it may at first seem:

> *The question is a tough one. Who does pick up the tab? In theory
> the taxpayer should. That is the most equitable approach, but it
> puts government in with both feet, maybe more than we would like.
> So we opt for a compromise. The insured public could pick up a
> portion of the costs of care for the poor and the near-poor. To what
> extent can the carriers stick their own policyholders with responsi-
> bility for the less fortunate and let the uninsured, or those who are
> not with them, go scot-free? That is a question we could debate
> endlessly.*
>
> Robert F. Froehlke

The tax questions are especially interesting for the broader issues they raise.
Unclear for now is how often state premium tax per se is an appreciable
impetus to self-insurance. Spencer doubts it is decisive:

> For years, the premium tax has been cited as the primary reason why
> employers self-insure their coverage. It is true that no employer wants to
> pay, directly or indirectly, a tax of 2 percent (the most common amount) on
> premiums—especially for insurance which is beneficial to society. In the
> final analysis, however, most employers will probably list reserves or total
> insurance company retention charges as the reason for self-insuring; pre-
> mium taxes usually rank further down the list.[25]

The Insurance Carrier's Retention

The insurance company retention charge, ranking high on Spencer's list
of employer concerns, contains different combinations of charges for claims
administration, contract administration, commissions, printing expenses, risk
charges, interest credits and charges, and contingency reserves, including
profit and amortization. Of these, profit and risk charges tend to stimulate the
liveliest discussion.

Profit

Within the retention, there is a charge for the commercial carrier's profit,
or in the case of the mutual companies and the service plans, a functional
equivalent of profit in operating gain, or overhead charges. Some critics of the
industry like to call attention to opulent glass skyscrapers, generous executive
salaries, and lavish image-building advertising as evidence of excess discre-
tionary money in the insurance business. For multiple line insurance firms, the
life and casualty business is said to contribute more towards skyscrapers and
the like than does health insurance. Spokesmen for the industry take issue with
the inference that their profits are excessive. For example, Thomas of the
Hancock:

> *There is a great deal of competition among all carriers and nonin-
> surance administrators in this area. If there ever was any surplus*

available for research and development into cost containment pos-
sibilities, competition has not permitted us to retain any. There
should have been R&D funds available; even 0.1 percent of pre-
miums over the years could have made the industry much more
effective in developing cost containment programs. The pressure
by major employers for low administrative costs or retentions has
not permitted the carriers to conduct adequate research.

                                                            Gordon W. Thomas

The themes that tend to run through these discussions are redolent of
Poor Richard's Almanac—you get what you pay for, spend money to save
money, and, despite the anachronism, another one worthy of Franklin:

Mr. Hickey has stated that as a consultant he has reduced retention
as low as 3 percent. We have set retention charges between 6–8
percent depending on the risk and reduced the bottom line from
12–50 percent. Let's look at the retention battle as if we haven't
reached the saturation point and reduce the 3 percent to 1 percent.
Isn't it fair to assume that if the caretakers of the funds were paid
next to nothing that they would do next to nothing? Solid cost
containment and administration has a price. The lowest bidder is
not always the best—I would not go to the moon on a rocket built by
the lowest bidder.

                                                            Robert B. Poitras

Few people in business object to someone making a fair profit and the issue of
profit may be more rhetorical than real.

Risk Charges

The carrier's risk charges are not easily isolated from the other components of the retention, but an analysis of his own firm's risk is an essential
element in the corporate manager's decision matrix. In the context of insurance, risk is a technical term with a precise meaning, and there are accounting
mechanisms by which the policyholder can assume specific segments of the
risk in order to reduce the carrier's risk charges. An example would be an
agreement in which the policyholder assumes the risk for a 90-day carryover
for claims that were incurred prior to the end of the contract year but were not
filed by the employee until after the new year began. This protects the carrier in
the event the contract were not renewed; the employer's risk in this illustration
would normally be relatively minor. Because of experience rating, the risk
charges rest chiefly on the assumption that the carrier will lose the account
when the current contract expires. Actually, for the very large cases, the
assumption seldom holds:

The very large employer is a sophisticated buyer of benefits who
has things pretty well pared down; he has clout and can usually get
his carrier to do his bidding. There is limited competition among

*the carriers for such an account because the employers are calling
the shots. Smaller companies do tend to change carriers more
frequently, in fact, insurance companies say that a major problem
with small cases is that they change too frequently. As a result, the
various acquisition costs which are important to any case—costs of
transfer, the cost of getting business and putting it on the books—
may not be properly recouped and this may cause overall prices to
be higher than they should be.*

Bruce F. Spencer

The ultimate assumption of risk occurs in self-funding, where the corporate entity takes on the entire risk of the health benefit plan, or all of it up to the level of a stop-loss policy. Some carriers argue that the gains from self-insuring the risk are negligible if the firm is realistic in its reckoning of where it stands:

*There is money to be saved on costs associated with insurance. But
it is erroneous to suggest that by not setting up outstanding claim
reserves through a carrier you can avoid reserves entirely. The
liability continues to exist; 20–25 percent of the annual premium
may be outstanding at any given point in time. The prudent corporation will reflect this liability on its balance sheet, just as it does if
it uses a Blue Cross plan or an insurance company. There can be
some savings on the investment of that money, but there are also
balancing costs. For example, when Deere and Company litigates a
claim, using staff lawyers or outside counsel, are those legal costs
charged against the health benefit cost center or do they show up as
legal expenses? Does the health benefit cost center get its share of
the depreciation of the building and office equipment, a share of
personnel department costs involved in hiring more people and
handling more turnover, and things like that? When firms go to
self-administration and self-insurance, they often think only of
direct costs—clerical help and maybe some share of computer
time—and lose sight of these other costs. Without very careful cost
accounting, a firm may lose money and not even know it.*

Michael P. McDonald

It should be pointed out here that some insurance companies—generally smaller ones—do not do the thorough cost accounting for their clients that McDonald is advocating self-insured firms undertake. The cash flow adjustments to which McDonald alludes are discussed below, under the rubric of reserves, the time value of money, and the devices the carrier develops to credit the policyholder for interest on reserves.

When the concept of risk is removed from the confines of the insurance business, it assumes added meaning from the standpoint of corporate strategy. Sieverts suggests that the narrow fiscal risk that the employer consciously accepts when he opts for self-funding may be inconsequential compared with the longer-range risk he may not even deliberately have decided he was willing to assume:

*There is an interesting kind of special risk built in for a corporation
whose money managers see the immediate gains that might be*

> *achieved by going to consulting firms and building a superstructure*
> *within their own corporation. Two or three years later, the money*
> *market might have changed totally, the tax structure might have*
> *gone through some radical revisions, and then you may find your-*
> *self with an equal temptation to go back to what you had before.*
> *But this is a tar baby phenomenon. It is rather easy to fire an*
> *insurance carrier. It is harder to fire your own operation in a*
> *situation like this, unless you are an extraordinarily flint-hearted*
> *employer, and there aren't very many of those around.*
>
> Steven Sieverts

By asking what will happen if the environment changes radically, Sieverts is essentially advocating a strategic planning exercise. Others in the
insurance industry marshal similar arguments against self-insurance.
McDonald of Blue Cross suggests that the state tax laws will change in such a
way that it will no longer be advantageous to self-insure; Thomas of the
Hancock suggests that ERISA will eventually be changed so as to effectively
wipe out the advantages of self-insurance. Ralson of the Prudential suggests in
chapter 9 that HMOs may eventually preempt self-insurance; and here it is
implied that a change in the money markets or the tax laws could constitute an
environmental change so radical as to leave the firm stuck to a bureaucratic tar
baby. Spencer makes similar predictions about national health insurance, and,
for example, counsels that 501(c)(9) trusts be set up for multiple purposes so
that the funds will remain accessible even if Congress enacts a national health
insurance plan that puts the trust out of reach for the purpose of paying health
benefits.[26]

One rebuttal to this general line of argument against self-insurance is the
solution third-party administrators seem to represent. A firm that self-funds the
benefit but contracts out its administration seems to avoid setting up Sieverts's
bureaucratic tar baby, waiting to be confronted a year or two down the road if
the national financing system for health care should change:

> *Doesn't the point argue just as well for an arrangement, not with an*
> *insurance carrier, but with a strictly administrative services firm*
> *that processes claims in a responsive, expeditious, and cost-*
> *effective way? Then if you are unsatisfied or if your circumstances*
> *change, you can terminate your contract with them after this or that*
> *year and switch. You then have the best of both worlds.*
>
> William J. Bicknell

Reserves and the Time Value of Money

The critical judgment with respect to reserves held by the carrier is how
much more these funds could otherwise be earning for the firm if invested in
the business or in the money markets:

> *You have to balance the cost of capital to the corporation against*
> *the interest credit or the equivalent of compensating the employer*

for the time value of the reserve money. What can the insurance companies do for you? Other than applying an interest rate to a reserve factor and crediting that back in a dividend formula, insurance companies can compensate you for the time value of reserve money through extending grace periods, adding retrospective premium adjustments, and so on.

Michael J. Gulotta

Reserves are held by the carrier to cover claims that are due but as yet unpaid; in the course of settlement; or incurred but as yet unreported. In self-funding the benefit and assuming responsibility for those claims, the employer obviates the carrier's reserve needs. To protect himself against fluctuations in claims, a self-funding employer may choose to establish his own reserves. But unlike the carrier the self-funding employer needs no protection against the contingency that he will unexpectedly terminate his own contract. As to both the level and the uses of funds held in reserve he will have considerably more latitude than did his carrier. This is generally accepted; the quotations in the box indicate that the consensus breaks down on the question of how much money—expressed as percentage of premium—is really at stake. Kaplan argues a strong case for self-funding, but others have trouble reconciling the figures he quotes with their own experiences.

There is no magic formula nor anything approaching unanimity on how to estimate the cost-saving potential of bringing the reserves and the risk in-house. Even the most optimistic concede this essential caveat: shaving percentage points off the 15 or 10 percent constituting administrative costs will be the height of folly if the exercise obscures the employer's sight of the other 85 or 90 percent of the premium. The important long-range costs are tied to the costs and volume of claims paid; success in monitoring those will be the litmus test.

Some one-time savings may be within grasp of many firms that have not yet streamlined to the maximum the financing of their health benefit plans. But the mechanisms now exist for achieving maximal savings in this area:

The major insurance carriers write around two-thirds of all the employee benefit plans privately insured. And 25 to 35 percent of all that business is already administrative services only, minimum premium, or derivations thereof. The majority have already eliminated or significantly reduced premium taxes, reserves, and much of the redundancy in the retention. That is 5 or 10 cents of the premium dollar. I submit that the other 90 cents of the premium dollar is where the action is.

Henry A. DiPrete

The remaining 90 or so cents of the premium dollar is inseparable from the health care delivery system. Extracting savings from this area is more complex and much less fully explored than the realm of administrative savings. The costs of claims themselves are the frontier, very much in need of the same joint creativity between industry and insurer that produced minimum premium plans, administrative services only contracts, and other financing and

SLICING THE PREMIUM PIE

Samuel X. Kaplan: If you self-insure you have the reserves to invest, and if you have a 501(c)(9) trust, you pay no taxes on that income. The insurance company has limits on where it can invest those reserves, and has to pay taxes on the investment income. By self-insuring you eliminate all the insurance company expenses and all premium taxes, plus you have cash flow on the reserves, you have the use of that money, and you have tax-free interest on that investment. Corporations can earn a lot more with those reserves than insurance companies could hope to do. From our experience with corporations that have self-insured, the savings are between 10 and 15 percent.

Thomas O. Pyle: I'm confused. It is true that reserves invested by insurance companies earn less than those same monies invested by commercial enterprises. Now you can invest the money in your business—say, tractors—or put it in the money market. Even very clever people can't put it in two places at once: either you have the reserves invested and earning the money or you have tractors, not both. If insurance companies can earn, say, 7 percent interest and zippy money managers working for commercial companies can earn 9 percent, there is a 2 percent spread. It has also been pointed out that the insurance companies pay taxes on those investments, although that is not true of all the insurance companies and certainly not the dominant insurer in the health field, Blue Cross. And it is also true that you can buy bonds and various forms of governmental securities to avoid paying taxes on investments. But let us assume the carrier pays a 50 percent tax—3.5 percent of the 7 percent. If I correctly understand what is being said, the money available to reduce premiums under the insurance company deal is 3.5 percent and the zippy money manager has reduced his premiums by 9 percent, which is a 5.5 percent difference before taxes. However, nobody is paying more than 5 percent for administrative services unless he is just a bad manager, so the total of those two things, worst case, is 10.5 percent, and I assume these people who sell administrative services like to earn profits and do not do it for free. I fail to see how you can get 15 percent out of any of these things unless you have been buying badly or unless you get into the other 90 percent, which is the health care side of it.

John Hickey: I agree. It is less than 10 percent. You have to take that 5.5 percent interest rate that you came down to and apply it to a reserve that is maybe only a quarter of a year's cost. That brings you down to an average of maybe 6 percent off the top. I cannot buy Mr. Kaplan's estimate of 10 or 15 percent difference off the top through premium taxes and cash flow advantages and the like. Once you get past the premium taxes and the potential interest on reserves, you are down to administrative expenses and who can administer the claims more cheaply. I doubt you can make up 10 percent there.

William J. Bicknell: There is, though, some substantial spread in the administrative expenses charged by carriers, third-party administrators, and the like.

Hickey: Sure, the potential for some savings is real. But it greatly depends on where you start and the real potential is available mainly to very large corporations, not to firms with under 500 employees. In large corporations total retention is probably in the neighborhood of 4 to 5 percent of claims. That includes premium taxes and also some credit for interest on reserves. I do think the hope of taking 10 or 15 percent off the top is unrealistic.

administrative innovations designed to reduce the corporate policyholder's costs:

> *The Blues and commercial carriers both feel a clear responsibility—a social responsibility and a political responsibility, the latter perhaps a little more selfish than the former. Because to the extent that we do not fulfill this responsibility and bring health care costs into line with the general economy, we know who will become deeply involved, and the prospect of a larger government role causes us grave concern.*
>
> Robert F. Froehlke

Using Claims Data to Contain Health Care Costs

The costs of an employee health benefit are like an iceberg: administrative service costs are the tip above the water, and paid claims the far more critical bulk hidden below the surface. In recent years, benefits managers have begun to reorient their attention from the administrative costs to the less obvious but much larger cost-saving potential represented in incurred claims. This shift is occurring because of the variable but shrinking and inevitably limited amounts of money remaining to be saved in the realm of administration of the benefit package, as discussed above, and because there are legions of recognized experts on whom a firm can call for advice—carriers, brokers, fee-paid consultants, third-party administrators, and other kinds of advisers.[27] Most large corporations now have in-house managers with the expertise needed to protect the corporation's interests and weigh the relative merits and risks of alternative funding arrangements. Having made such an assessment, implementation is relatively straightforward; it is a matter of locating the carrier or administrator offering the best package and entering into a contract. The effector arms are easy to identify.

Influencing the Costs of Claims

When he starts to explore the hidden part of the iceberg comprising the costs of paid claims, the benefits manager is much harder pressed to find appropriate effector arms directed toward cost containment. Insurance carriers have tended to work on the relatively noncontroversial aspects of paying claims, and have developed considerable expertise in verifying the legitimacy of claims for medical care services already rendered. (Even this basic insurance carrier service has often been foregone by management in the name of placid labor relations.) Among the more sophisticated and important of the carriers' efforts to contain the costs of claims are programs to coordinate benefits.

Coordination of Benefits

Coordination of benefits (COB) programs can achieve some savings for corporate policyholders, but do so by identifying duplicative coverage, and not by reviewing the utilization of services with an eye toward preventing inappropriate or unwarranted use. COB addresses the volume of *claims*; its effect on the volume of *services* is indirect and probably negligible. The savings potential of COB was recently dramatized in the Borden case:[28]

> Borden saved over 14 percent in COB, but this is an extreme case. They were coordinating against things like no-fault, which some insurance companies don't do, or do less effectively, and against Workers' Compensation—that is, in realms that have largely been ignored for one reason or another. Other companies really wanting to put their attention to COB could increase their savings by looking at all these various possibilities and by being stringent. But I think 14 percent is probably about as far as you'll ever see anybody go, and a lot farther than most will go.
>
> Bruce F. Spencer

Some other experiences with COB were touched on in the first volume of this series.[29] For example, Standard Oil of California reported to a survey of the Washington Business Group on Health that COB saved the firm $18.6 million in 1973, $22.6 million in 1974, and $32 million in 1975.[30] Equitable Life estimated in 1976 that the aggregate COB savings potential for all carriers nationwide is close to $1 billion annually.[31] But there are limits on how much coordination of benefits can save a firm because the program lacks direct impact on the volume of services delivered, the cost of those services, or their appropriateness.

Health Maintenance Organizations

By contrast, HMOs represent an approach with potential for altering the delivery system in the direction of utilization control. Effective HMOs achieve their results by reducing the use of inappropriate or unnecessary services and by establishing a management structure for health services delivery. Closed panel plans like Kaiser have well-established histories of successfully lowering hospital rates; some of the newer generations of individual practice association (IPA)-HMOs, or "fee-for-service HMOs," are beginning to demonstrate that they can implement peer review programs with proper incentives that reduce hospital days per thousand members. The Minneapolis experience[32] is a widely quoted recent example. Published accounts of HMO performance suggest that the unstructured fee-for-service health care system makes greater use of inpatient hospital care than is necessary, or even beneficial. This evidence has led several large corporations to explore the feasibility of sponsoring or catalyzing the development of HMOs in communities where none exist, to serve concentrations of employees of the firm and their families. The fifth volume in the Industry and Health Care series explored this emerging trend.[33] For any of several reasons, many corporations are unable to actively promote HMO growth, or are confronted with such unfavorable local situations that chances of success are remote. These corporations are actively seeking other mechanisms for analyzing and ultimately influencing the appropriate use of health care services financed through their employee benefit plans. The experience of fee-for-service HMOs points to utilization review as an important mechanism to consider, especially where the closed financial system of a prepaid plan is an unrealistic short-term goal.

Health Services Data for Utilization Review

From the corporate manager's perspective the meaning of the term *utilization review* is changing as more effective uses of health care data are being found. For example, an array of diagnostic and treatment procedures related to individual providers and patients provides a broad screen in which to catch gross overutilization or misuse. In some instances, multiple and repeated injections or treatments stand out as beyond the broad band of acceptable medical practice. In others, hospital lengths of stay are far outside accepted standards. Both examples could provide the substratum for an information campaign directed at a change in the behavior of provider or patient, or both. A form of utilization review with much greater potential for cost savings, but one that is much more complex to administer, occurs when the group responsible for claims administration seeks to enlist medical leadership in an effort to identify and eliminate lesser degrees of overuse—in effect to compress the wide band of medically accepted practice—through a process of rigorous peer review and peer pressure backed up by an effective administrative system.

A Problem Is Where to Begin

Awareness of the possibilities of using health care data has led to a groundswell of demand from corporations for their insurance carriers to provide meaningful utilization data that they can examine and "massage." Carriers have tended to respond by emphasizing the costs of generating new data and questioning the wisdom of amassing data for its own sake without knowing exactly how it is to be used.

Always the criticism is why don't you do more. If we're giving 100 percent we should give 400 percent. The problem is that cost containment costs money. So we, as carriers, must have a very, very open dialogue with our customers about what their needs are and what they want us to do. Because when we start pulling this material together and refusing claims or whatever—intervening in the delivery system as we're calling it here—we had better have our customer alongside or we will fail.

Joseph W. Mullen, Jr.

These concerns give rise to a kind of chicken-and-egg debate. Some corporate policyholders are demanding data from their carriers, feeling that without the data in hand and a better feel for both the exact nature and scope of the utilization problems they may face and the range of workable solutions within their grasp, they cannot predict what corrective measures the data might support. But the carriers are unconvinced that a major investment in data collection is justified unless the firms requesting more information have a plan to use it:

A lot of people are interested in having data, but I hope before this goes too far that we develop an organized plan to use the data that has a reasonable probability of success. For example, in Blue Shield we have a number of coding systems in our plans around this country, and we have looked at the cost of implementing a uniform coding system for all Blue Shield plans. It's millions of dollars. I worry that if we don't have an organized plan with a probability of success, are we just creating data for people who want to do research? That may be interesting, but it may not be a justifiable expenditure. We should be very careful before proceeding along those lines; there should be some real-world utility in what is being asked for.

Michael P. McDonald

Some are totally unsympathetic with this argument, which they consider a mere smokescreen:

You make a case for nonuniform data on the grounds that we're not absolutely sure we can do anything with more uniform data. Granted, it's absurd to collect reams of data with no thought in mind of what to do. But to make the case for nonuniform data nationally, you really make the case for precluding any kind of assessment of what's going on, any kind of planning for alternative intervention, any kind of evaluation of alternative strategies. I think that's an extraordinarily destructive case you're making; a case for extreme inaction, cleverly stated.

William J. Bicknell

But corporate policyholders face analogous challenges in allocating their resources internally. Wineland of Armco describes these complexities (p. 37) and the need to avoid going down blind alleys:

PUTTING DATA TO WORK

Stephen C. Caulfield: Our system begins with total aggregated data of the whole health system, nationwide, then gradually disaggregates by diagnosis, by procedure, by region, and so forth and then makes comparisons that show us where we have problems. The objective is to develop data with which to manage an orderly system, not to engage in rascal hunting for its own sake.

Samuel X. Kaplan: We've been able to prove that cost containment and quality of care go hand in hand. When you discover doctors overutilizing and cut down on that, you improve the quality of care. When you discover treatments that are being rendered unnecessarily and do away with that, you are enhancing quality. And at the same time, when you're doing effective utilization review, you can pick up the doctors who are underutilizing and can take action against them too.

Willis B. Goldbeck: There's another whole class of data that's not particularly sensational but that can help a consumer make an informed decision. For example, three major hospitals in Washington, D.C., charged for the identical procedure fees differing by over $100. The average patient who goes to a surgeon in the city has a choice among those hospitals since many surgeons have admitting privileges at all three. So, given the right incentives, that noncontroversial hospital cost data could influence a patient's decision, if it were made available in a straightforward and timely way.

Thomas O. Pyle: The problem with that, as you well know, is that the incentives are not right. We need to distinguish between data to predict and data to control. Predictive data is nice, but I'm convinced that the kind of data we need to control—to make policy decisions five years out—could be put together, seat-of-the-pants fashion, right now. The question is whether people are willing to bite the bullet and to exert the leverage that's necessary, to change the structure of benefits, change provider and consumer behavior, change capital investments, and so on. I don't see what good all of the data are going to do without the commitment to confront these difficult issues.

John L. Brown: About two years ago Genesco reshaped our data system so that we can capture our operating experiences by location. After about a year and a half, we took this information to our carrier and mutually agreed on a plan of action that had the carrier approach the providers who stood out as overutilizers, while we undertook a rather ambitious educational program aimed toward the employees in the affected locations. Within eight months, we saw a more than 50 percent reduction of hospital utilization in the areas identified as problems. These were areas where our loss ratio was running as high as 150 to 175 percent, compared with an average across Tennessee of 60 to 70 percent. Where our loss ratio is 90 percent or less we simply monitor our experience. In areas identified as hot spots through these loss ratios, we look at diagnoses, by physician and by procedure, and compare those with local, regional, and national norms. We're now extending this program into Mississippi and Alabama and in each case we've been able to get the data we need to do this. Another program we've recently implemented is coordination of benefits. We now return the claims charge lists to each of our locations and ask the personnel directors there to go over the detailed physician's bill or hospital invoice with the employee who was treated, just to make certain that the employee really did receive the services for which we paid. I know a company in Florida that has been doing this for the last three years and they are absolutely sure that it saves them a minimum of 10 percent of premium. Our program is too new to evaluate, but in the first month one of the plants did identify a $3,000 error. I think these are some pretty good examples of what can be done with currently existing data.

There's another little complexity here. A corporation like Armco cannot act unilaterally to expand its compensation program. The union is involved. Typically, when management suggests a change, say an ambulatory care benefit or a second opinion program, the union's retort is, "Fine. If you want that, what are you offering us in return?" So there is a cost. Then, to further complicate matters, we're not even sure that ambulatory care or second opinion surgery will effect a cost savings to the corporation, so now we have to barter for something in which we have little confidence. Frankly, I'm not too anxious to do that. As a benefits manager, I'm going to be cautious. The risk is too great. If I go off and plow new ground, it costs me not only administrative dollars to collect the data, and so forth, but real dollars to compensate the union, and I may not get any return in the end. Corporate benefits people must have more conclusive data before we can act. I go to management and say I need people and resources to develop data to save money in the health care area, and they ask what money I am going to save. I say I don't know, I need the data to answer that, It looks like I'm chasing my tail, and management is understandably reluctant to invest computer money on a health data processing system that may work, and may supply useful data. Until I can come back with a

*more conclusive plan, they would rather put in an inventory track-
ing system or a raw materials purchase control that will work.
Meanwhile, I have reams of IBM paper from our carriers, with data
they provide in their system, and their format, needing to be con-
verted to a form we can use. This is a long, involved process, that
takes money and resources, and we find ourselves with a classic
chicken-and-egg problem.*

David C. Wineland

Wineland's labor relations concerns are a real constraint for many firms.
There is, however, much common ground on which labor and management can
meet and pursue cost-containment in health. Such areas of mutual interest
were recently identified in a collection of position papers, covering the gamut
of health care cost containment strategies, published by an informal organization of major labor and management leaders called the Labor Management
Group.[34]

The practical issues Wineland raises demonstrate again that the second-
order question of implementation—of what is to be done with the data through
what effector arms—is inseparable from and in some ways antecedent to the
first-order question of what data firms should ask their carriers to generate. The
quotations in the box (pp. 36–37) address this two-part data need.

A Taft-Hartley Multi-Employer Trust as a Management System

The United Mine Workers of America Health and Retirement Funds and
the United Storeworkers Security Plan, whose programs are outlined in part III,
illustrate the use of claims data not only to monitor the utilization of services,
but gradually to alter practices. As Caulfield points out in his report (chapter
12), the Mine Workers' system was implemented for less than a full year before
the Health and Retirement Funds were restructured in the 1978 wage
agreements that culminated a 110-day strike. However, the design and testing
of the system was a valuable learning experience, and many of the concepts on
which it rested are applicable across the board. A basic premise was that
meaningful data can have important persuasive power:

*When we began to develop our data system in 1974 we made a very
strong effort to include the kinds of questions practicing physicians
in our regions would want answered. The physician practicing
alone or in a group has relatively little data about his practice in
comparison with others, and by and large is keenly interested in
these kinds of things. As a strategy for using data to effect change, it
is possible to engage the physician's professional interest simply by
demonstrating how his practice deviates from various "norms." On
the employer side, the data are likewise useful for eliciting interest
in the problem of cost containment and health benefits management and in beginning to create an atmosphere in the workplace
conducive to health promotion. This is a complicated problem that
cannot be solved by the provider and employer alone; the employee must also be involved. We talk about corporations saving*

money, but rarely talk about passing those savings on to the employee. The attributes of a successful health insurance program from the employee's perspective are three: let me go where I want to go, pay the doctor promptly, and do not reject any claims. And the corresponding attributes for management, or a managed system, are the opposite: to manage the markets, you cannot let employees have total free choice, to pay claims responsibly you must review third-party liabilities, coordination of benefits, level of benefits, fee acceptability, and duplicate payments. These reviews take time and if done properly lead to some level of rejected claims. Unless there are some incentives that flow to the employee, it will be very difficult to engage their interest in this process of managing the system. The corporation must be willing to share some of the savings with employees as an incentive for cost control.

Stephen C. Caulfield

To some extent, the Mine Workers' and Storeworkers' programs described in part III of this volume may serve as models for other self-funded plans, but as multi-employer trusts, under the Taft-Hartley Act, they are constrained to operate within a prenegotiated fixed budget, and therefore differ importantly from the benefit plans provided by most individual employers.

Typically, the Taft-Hartley trusts (some 4,800 plans in 1973, representing less than 4 percent of all group health insurance plans) exist in multi-employer situations, for example in service, coal mining, construction, apparel, and casual employment.[35] The most common pattern of bargaining in these cases is to negotiate prospectively, for the duration of the collective bargaining agreement, a fixed contribution from the signatory companies (usually a certain number of cents per hour, a set percentage of the payroll or an amount reflecting rates of productivity, such as coal tonnage in the mining industry). The level of income to the fund is thus determined by the wage agreement, and unanticipated expenses or shortages in expected contributions can force cuts in the benefit package. Certainly labor feels stronger incentives to control health care costs in plans with a finite employer contribution than in those where the employment contract guarantees a certain level of benefits regardless of cost. Often there is also a different attitude toward the program on the part of employees who tend to think of a health and welfare fund as their plan and are more willing to share in cost containment ideas and to accept administrative fiats. Employees covered by a single-employer plan have been more likely to view it as the employers plan and less inclined to want to join with management in efforts to save money.

Multi-employer trusts are among the principal clients of Samuel X. Kaplan's U.S. Administrators, described in chapter 11. But his firm also provides some corporate clients, in the western part of the country, a claims review system that intervenes in the medical care process to decrease the use of both hospital and ambulatory services when they exceed medical standards. To what degree Kaplan's approach is generalizable to the situations of other employers in other parts of the country remains to be seen. Skeptics believe that Kaplan "gets away with" his adversary role because his organization is relatively small (handling claims for about 400,000 employees). Admirers argue that as U.S. Administrators' share of the market grows, the firm should become even more effective. The debate over the Kaplan system is important for its implications—affirmative and negative—concerning immediate and long-range possibilities of controlling health care costs in the unstructured fee-for-service medical system financed through conventional reimbursement insurance.

U.S. Administrators: "A Slugfest with Providers"

Either there will be a slugfest with providers or else employers will go on writing blank checks—where are the controls on the current system? Insurance companies don't have the guts to take the bull by the horn and do real claims control.

Samuel X. Kaplan

U.S. Administrators is based in Los Angeles, California, and originated as an administrator of prepaid drug plans. The firm now also provides administrative services for hospital and medical/surgical plans and dental plans, also prescription drug and vision plans and workers' compensation and handles an annual load of about $74,532,000 in claims. Kaplan's system uses computerized "model treatment screens" to review every claim. The computer program makes all the routine checks on eligibility conducted by conventional carriers, checks fees against computerized fee profiles, and, in addition, compares the treatment ordered for the specific diagnosis against a model treatment plan that Kaplan has developed for groups of diseases in the International Classification of Diseases Adapted (ICDA) code book:

> *Our model treatment screens take every diagnosis—3,400 odd—and establish all the treatments that might reasonably be encountered for each one and with what frequency—how many return visits to the physician, how many lab tests of what sort, how much x-ray, and so on.*

In concept, the review against preestablished standards resembles the approach of professional standards review organizations (PSROs), but U.S. Administrators is in effect conducting a PSRO-type review on every medical encounter (both ambulatory and inpatient hospital care) falling within its purview. Kaplan asserts that his system, like PSROs, relies on respected medical practitioners to set the standards of care:

> *We put together a group we call a Council of Health Professionals— twenty-three outstanding physicians, surgeons, dentists, all members of their professional societies, all highly respected practitioners with part-time teaching positions at major educational institutions. They sat down and hammered out these model treatment screens for each diagnosis and then they went back to their specialty societies for additional input.*

Hospital lengths of stay are in general set at the seventy-fifth percentile of the professional activity study (PAS) for different regions, as determined by the Commission on Hospital and Professional Activities (CHPA). Some variations may be acceptable in the model treatment profiles, and the medical director can further ease the guidelines if in his judgment such an action is warranted. Ambulatory standards are set without the benefit of a national data base like the CHPA's, but represent the informed opinion of a medical panel. A striking departure from PSROs is the manner in which U.S. Administrators applies its standards:

> Every claim is subjected to the model treatment screen. Charges are checked against our computerized fee profiles and are disallowed if excessive. On hospital stays, we screen every miscellaneous charge. These now constitute about 50 percent of hospital bills, and they are largely ignored by the usual claims review. We also monitor length of stay. When a patient is admitted to the hospital, the admittance office calls us to confirm coverage and benefit level, whereupon we ask for the admitting diagnosis and advise the hospital of the length of stay we are authorizing. That night, our computer automatically writes a letter to the attending physician with a length of stay allowance. If the diagnosis were appendicitis, for example, the letter would specify: "no surgery, three days; surgery, five days; any further length of stay, you justify it." We put the doctor on notice. "If you leave that patient in an extra day without justification, you will pay for it. We will not pay for it nor will the patient." Copies of this letter go to the hospital and the patient, who is told to notify us immediately if he receives a bill. We'll use any kind of threat we can think of—letters to medical or dental societies, letters and calls to the local newspaper or the local TV and radio stations if we have to . . . whatever it takes. But I'll tell you something, you can get better quality care for your people this way for a lot less money.

About one-third of the claims are caught in Kaplan's computer screens and are processed first through a lay claims handler. Questions go to the medical director, and sometimes on up for final arbitration to the Council of Health Professionals:

> It's not a lay person calling an anesthesiologist onto the carpet. When there's a dispute, an anesthesiologist calls an anesthesiologist. That's an important difference because the seeming severity of the case is usually the justification offered for a higher fee or a longer hospital stay, and that's a medical judgment.

Kaplan asserts that he achieves cost savings in the neighborhood of 10 to 30 percent using the model treatment profile. He shrugs off the physician antipathy occasioned by the program on grounds that the displeased physicians are "abusers," who are out of the mainstream of medicine:

> The majority of these guys aren't abusers. That's important to remember. Most are doing a decent job. It's the minority we're after, and they're hurting the whole profession.

Kaplan offers the growth in his business as evidence that he is serving a real need:

> Sure, we may scare off some physicians who may decide it's not worth their while to treat patients who are in our programs. But if this were a serious problem we wouldn't be getting the business we have. Our volume has increased 40 percent compounded annually over the last five years and that's about a 50-50 mix between union and nonunion groups. I think we're doing something right, and others must think so too.

The Carriers Respond

It comes as no surprise that the insurance industry fails to share Kaplan's enthusiasm for his approach to the problem of health care costs. They find it far too radical and fear that its widespread adoption would lead to acrimony among providers:

> Mr. Kaplan's system certainly does get the doctors' attention. That's basically what it is about. I would suggest that if the Blues and the commercial carriers did what he does as a planned program, we would not only get their attention, we would set up an adverse situation. I believe that no cost containment program or national health insurance plan can succeed without the cooperation of the providers. I firmly believe that the doctors are hearing us and are coming around.
>
> Robert F. Froehlke

Also, the carriers feel, Kaplan's approach, on a wide scale, would lack support from the public because it would inconvenience patients:

> We are looking for incremental change, over time, in how physicians practice. Public opinion polls repeatedly show most consumers are quite well satisfied with their own care. There are very serious limits to how far one can go on a large scale in trying to intervene in the name of consumers who do not want that intervention. Perhaps small plans, union plans, can go out and engage in the kind of aggressive behavior described here and get away with it for a while. But if that were tried on a larger scale, I think it might create tremendous backlash, not only from the providers, but from the consumers.
>
> Steven Sieverts

In the past, employers have demanded and carriers have provided conciliatory and expeditious processing of medical claims; conflict was studiously avoided:

> Our customers, to whom we make utilization data available, are extremely cautious. There are numerous legal and labor relations

issues to be considered, and they go through a very deliberate well-thought-out, and well-communicated process before they act.
Joseph W. Mullen, Jr.

An important question is whether the cost problem is yet severe enough to alter this fundamental approach. Some believe so:

In the face of a stuttering economy and at best a very unsure economic outlook in this country, Allied Chemical has a very real concern with medical insurance cost increases. In 1965 we spent $29 million for medical insurance, sick leave, and workers' compensation. By the end of 1978 it will be closer to $55 million, or about an 83 percent increase. I want to know where the potential for cost savings is. Our company is probably typical of much of major industry today. We are awakening to the fact that the barn is burning, and we really don't see or expect any near-term help from the providers or the carriers. We think we have to move forward on our own and develop the kinds of data and systems needed to make decisions. Mr. Kaplan may represent an extreme on one end, but I very frankly feel that the other extreme is represented by the carriers and the providers. Meanwhile we project our costs in this arena, if left unchallenged, to be at about $150 million ten years from now. That rate of increase is simply unacceptable to our company, and I think to industry in general.
Albert F. Ritardi

From the likes of Allied Chemical, the insurance industry, both commercial and nonprofit, now faces a basic challenge. Pressures are on them to supply more and better data to satisfy at least two distinct needs emerging from the newer and more involved employee benefits manager. Corporations want baseline utilization data profiling providers and patients, in time perhaps to serve effective claims review systems but for now at least to allow them to pinpoint where their problems are. In addition, they will want specialized data on a variety of experimental cost containment programs so that they can evaluate these systematically and build toward long-range solutions to the problem of health care costs. A current example of an experimental program requiring a special data collection effort is second surgical opinion, discussed in the box.

The United Mine Workers' experience suggests that the short-term and longer range data needs are complementary:

As soon as our data system was up and running we were approached by academic researchers, for example a group wishing to use our data in a study of the use of oxygen therapy in treating chronic obstructive pulmonary disease. They use our data base for their research, which is blind to us. We don't intervene at all, but simply provide specific data they request. The research program reimburses the funds for all costs related to generating data. I think it's important not to lose sight of that longer term payoff. Everyone talks about the poor quality of medical claims data, that diagnoses are distorted, that procedures are not fully reported, that it's

DATA TO MONITOR
SECOND SURGICAL OPINION

David H. Winkworth: We at Mobil Oil instituted six changes in our plan last July: second surgical opinion, ambulatory surgical care, extended care facilities, home health care agencies, outpatient testing, and alcohol and drug abuse rehabilitation facilities. We did it without elegant data, since little was available. One of our problems now is getting our plan administrator to give us data on what's happening with the new programs. Management is going to be asking for an accounting in a year or so, and unless we get some good hard data, we're going to have problems in responding.

Joseph W. Mullen, Jr.: Let me respond to that, since we're the carrier in question. Metropolitan's position on second surgical opinion is that we have suspended judgment. We don't know whether it is cost effective, so we are suggesting to our corporate clients that we experiment together in this area. Several clients have elected to do that, and they are the forward-looking firms right now. As an experimental program, it is being treated specially. We don't expect quick answers; it will take three to five years and an investment into a very particular measuring system to ascertain whether the program is cost effective. We must track those who sought a second opinion for several years before we can start forming some conclusions. Our enthusiasm is tempered by that real-world constraint.

Richard H. Egdahl: But do you have it so rigged that after three to five years Mobil's management will be able to decide definitively whether to discontinue the program or keep it going?

Mullen: The program is so designed that after three to five years we will have collected enough data to judge whether it is cost effective.

Lesley L. Ralson: We've been doing an experimental program for Prudential employees in New Jersey for two years. I have no conclusive proof, but a strong suspicion that second surgical opinion *is* cost effective. We'd like to believe we've seen quality improvement as a result of the program and I think we can justify on that basis alone, with the idea that there will be some savings later on.

Egdahl: But will you be collecting the kind of data that you can share with your corporate clients and allow them to track their own experiences with you?

Ralson: First we need to share the data with the American College of Surgeons and the New Jersey College of Surgeons before we publish it. We have found that an agreement of this nature is essential in order to get the medical community's cooperation.

Arthur G. Carty: It does very little good to simply offer second surgical opinion and then sit back to see what happens. You've got to be willing to put in a lot of work bringing patients and providers along to understand and participate in these programs.

Henry A. DiPrete: That is true of most changes in benefit plan design. There is no point in making these changes if you don't bother to convince providers and patients to make the requisite changes in their practices and attitudes. Sometimes these innovations just get popped into the plan almost on whim, and then they tend either not to be used at all, or not to be used appropriately.

Willis B. Goldbeck: One of the problems all over the country is the rather low participation rates in these experimental programs, but a group of companies in a given community could correct this problem. Why not make the second opinion mandatory? There's no inherent reason not to; it is no denial of the employee's rights to require that he have a second opinion, so long as he is given absolute freedom to choose which opinion to act on. If the employers in a given community come to such an understanding, it would certainly speed up the data collection process, and our ability to measure the true value of the second opinion concept.

difficult to code, that it's vague. I grant all that. But it's possible to maximize what we get from the claims payment process. We need standardized data and some agreement about what data ought to be captured. There is no need to drown ourselves in printouts. We should simply catch the information that we can get and count it uniformly, and then make that data base available for two purposes—short-term management and long-term academic research into fundamental issues of quality and efficacy of care.
Stephen C. Caulfield

Once they possess the utilization data necessary for Caulfield's short-term management, employers are likely to intensify their search for effective control systems—the effector arms that are as yet inadequately developed.

Where Are the Effector Arms?

Kaplan's model treatment profiles permit far less latitude in medical practice than remains in reviews conducted by Blue Shield physician panels, commercial carriers, and most, if not all, PSROs. The effectiveness of PSROs as a cost containment vehicle is in doubt; indeed, physician leadership in the PSRO movement is divided on the question of whether control of costs is essential to PSROs' primary mission of quality assurance.[36] Even where control of costs is an avowed goal, PSROs have little direct incentive to push to the margins of acceptable practice, and their performance to date reflects this:

> *Although I do not favor Mr. Kaplan's approach and feel that incremental change is the way we must go, I'm not all that satisfied with PSROs either. I don't think that they have done the job they should do. On the other hand, I don't think the carriers are a satisfactory replacement for them.*
>
> Lesley L. Ralson

Proponents of HMOs consider them the most satisfactory alternative because they restructure the incentives on physicians and put them at financial risk for their decisions. When it has become clear to participating physicians that they must alter their ordering practices to ensure the solvency of the plan, some HMOs have instituted very rigorous peer review along the lines of U.S. Administrators. But physicians' motivations to contain costs, even within the confines of an HMO, are not as uncomplicated as those of a third-party administrator.

In theory, the insurance carriers are motivated on behalf of their clients to keep costs down, to the extent that this is what their clients really want. Carriers are only beginning to feel a changing mandate, and it is by no means unambiguous. In addition, a practical handicap shared by the commercial carriers and the local Blue Cross and Blue Shield plans is a lack of concentration except in a very few geographical areas. In most local medical markets no one carrier has a sufficient share of the market to build a comprehensive data base or exercise unassailable influence:

> *We do develop profiles for clients of the Hancock, but these profiles are probably miniscule within any given geographic area and for any given provider. Except where we have a very large client who is a major force within an area, the amount of data that we can collect on any given provider is de minimus. We may have a fair amount of data on several routine procedures, but for the great bulk of procedures, we don't have enough data to negotiate vigorously with the providers and that is why we believe that it would be highly desirable to have available collective health data.*
>
> Gordon W. Thomas

The need for collective action serves as one argument against self-insurance:

> *I would submit that system intervention is much better accomplished by consolidating power rather than fragmenting it. An*

employer vying, by itself, with the hospital system in a particular area scarcely has the power that several employers using an insurance company could have. I'm not saying that anybody has done a good job of system intervention and I'm setting aside the HMO option which is really a different issue. I don't think that setting up a claims department in a corporation that may represent 10 percent of the people hospitalized in an area is going to have the same whack that several employers in that area could have by getting together and putting pressure on Blue Cross to do some things with the hospitals. I think it's paring down the power.

Thomas O. Pyle

But consolidation of power can also be viewed as a liability:

When you have a consolidation of power in the hands of one third party, can it really take the risk of pulling that trigger? There is a strong case for having several modest-sized levers or guns so that they can in fact be used. If you overconsolidate in a few very large third parties, it is very hard to do anything because there are so many secondary consequences—political, employment, and social, not to mention conflicting pressures from constituents: "Some of our clients want us to do this; some want us to do that; after all, you're only 30,000 employees, we can't really respond just to you" and so on. Some balance is needed because concentration of power is a two-edged sword.

William J. Bicknell

If geographic concentration helps, it appears to be less than the full answer:

I believe we are overemphasizing the advantages of aggregation of purchasing power. In the Appalachian corridor we represent perhaps 40 percent of the market, yet even there it is quite difficult to have an effective aggregated purchasing program. Aggregation of purchasing power doesn't guarantee cost savings particularly in an environment of limited competition.

Stephen C. Caulfield

When it comes to concentration of power, the Blue Cross and Blue Shield plans seem to have at least a potential advantage over any one of the commercial carriers, because they write about 40 to 45 percent of all job-related health insurance. The remainder is carved up among 1,000 or so commercial carriers, although the top twenty firms account for over 70 percent of the premium volume.[37] Variability in local Blues plans diminishes the aggregate influence they should theoretically have, but the Blues view both their market share and their local base as major selling points.

The commercial carriers are prevented by antitrust law from pooling their data resources, even for cost containment purposes, since those data might be used for price fixing (see chapter 15). The Health Insurance Association of America has been working to persuade Congress to enact an antitrust exemption for data collaboration in pursuit of health care cost containment. The size of the shadow cast by antitrust law is debated, as in the box, but there seems to

THE SWORD OF DAMOCLES: ANTITRUST

Richard H. Egdahl: The unavoidable question is why the carriers haven't pooled their claims data, developed uniform reporting systems, and implemented effective utilization review.

Robert F. Froehlke: I don't like the answer I have to give because I agree that such cooperation is a terrific idea. But if health insurance companies were to discuss working together to develop aggregate data, I'll guarantee that the Justice Department, the FTC, and the various committees of Congress would be on top of us in an instant for violating antitrust. The ends don't justify the means. It is just as illegal to act in concert to achieve the objective of holding costs down as it is to act in concert to raise prices. And if you look at the assets in the insurance industry, as many judges would do, the fines would be horrendous. We can't act in concert today. It will take an act of Congress to give us a waiver before we can collaborate to contain costs.

Willis B. Goldbeck: As a corollary to asking their carriers to do more, I wonder if employers are willing to go to bat for the carriers in securing an antitrust exemption from the government. If not, is it because the employers don't think the carriers should have such an exemption, or is it that they don't accept the carriers' contention that antitrust is a sufficient problem to warrant an exemption? It is my impression from recent meetings with the FTC and others that as more and more employers become self-funded and increasingly take on the role of insurance carriers, someone is going to decide that they too are subject to these antitrust laws. This possibility may even now be a developing incentive on the part of large employers to support some kind of blanket exemption for cost containment in health. Many people feel the administration is being inconsistent in asking hospitals to cut back, cooperate, share and institute all these marvelous voluntary cost containment programs, while the FTC is threatening to sue everybody that does any of the above. I would suggest that this is not an inconsistency on the part of the administration at all, but rather the result of two governmental bodies following their respective legislative mandates to the letter, exactly as we would want them to do, because to do otherwise would be to violate the mission Congress established for them. We, the voting public, should be giving the administration and Congress a collective message about which value we consider most important.

Bruce F. Spencer: I disagree. I think we are seeing another case of government agencies overstepping their legislative mandates, just as we saw in the implementation of ERISA, in tax code interpretations, and in a number of other instances. Sometimes, in fact, the legislature has had to step in and attempt to correct such a government agency. I'm not prepared to sit back and accept the idea that the FTC is really acting on its legislative mandate.

Steven Sieverts: Ultimately, Congress may indeed decide that the FTC has gone beyond its legislative mandate. But for now what the FTC and Congress hears from the public is to do more about health care costs not less. If business and industry want to see a shift, perhaps to see Congress pulling the reins on an FTC gone wild, then by all means, somebody must convey that message to them along with the insurance carriers, who are already asking for some kind of exemption to do a more effective job in health insurance.

Gilbert S. Omenn: Do large employers perceive a need for Congress to enact this FTC exemption for the insurance industry?

Albert F. Ritardi: I believe that it is a problem of such magnitude that we must bring the management of it to a higher level of sensitivity and awareness.

Judith K. Miller: I've talked enough with carriers to know that they feel very much reined in by the threat of antitrust action from the FTC. However, I'm not hearing an outpouring from this group about the need for Congressional action to loosen those reins.

Spencer: The real question is what each employer can do, and that doesn't require a comprehensive national data base. The employer's concern is what is happening to his premium, and because one firm's plan is different from another's, and the geographic locations are diverse the influences will be different. I'm not convinced that the employer cares terribly about the fact that the carrier with whom he happens to be insured has 0.2 percent of the entire insured population; for him the important point is who has 100 percent of his insured population.

Stephen C. Caulfield: Antitrust is a significant problem, and I certainly don't hold myself out to be an expert in the area. However, I do think that the insurance industry could reach an agreement to count things the same way without running any risk of antitrust constraints. One of the serious data problems

> we are facing is the fact that we haven't been able to reach an agreement about how to count things. We are not collecting uniform data. We don't code procedures consistently. We are moving that way on diagnoses, but we still have about five major procedure coding systems operative in this country. There is a real lack of consistency and uniformity about what kind of data we collect and how rigorously we require that data. It's difficult to aggregate data that are defined inconsistently.
>
> **Froehlke:** Again, that sounds fine, but our lawyers would say, why do you want to have this uniform system? What are you going to do with the data? If we respond that we're going to use it to negotiate with the providers to lower health care costs, our lawyers would warn us that we are running a very grave risk.

be little doubt that a shadow is indeed cast. At least for the present, there seem to be some real problems with carrier collaboration on the use of data for utilization review.

Looking to the Future

Granting the barriers to collective action, what is to prevent insurance companies as individual units from carrying out utilization review on the claims information they have? They receive all the data elements necessary for this activity in the claim forms submitted by providers. The insurance industry offers several explanations for the lack of strong, effective utilization review. First, most carriers either do not enter all information from the claims form into their computers, or do so only in a form that makes it very difficult to withdraw and array for utilization review. Second, there are real costs associated with the addition of information to their computer systems, which are customized for rapid processing for certification of eligibility and coordination of benefits and accurate payment of claims. Third, carrier programs for utilization review would have to be written and standards developed, similar to Kaplan's model treatment profiles, for each diagnosis and treatment procedure, both inpatient and ambulatory or for a systematically selected subset of the most common or most frequently questioned. Fourth, and probably most critical and difficult, a procedure would have to be activated to investigate each procedure captured in the computer screens, and to apply aggressive peer pressure on providers deviating from the standards without a satisfactory explanation of extenuating circumstances. Only after completing all these steps would a claims administrator have the necessary tools for effective utilization review. Over and above the financial costs of completing these steps, other risks have discouraged insurance companies and other groups from entering this new arena.

The primary hesitation is the fact that aggressive utilization review not infrequently creates an adversary situation between claims administrators and providers. An administrative firm with the exclusive purpose of processing claims accurately, efficiently, and cost effectively has a vastly different perspective on provider overutilization than does a large multiple line insurance company whose corporate mission traditionally has been to maintain public trust—in part by avoiding controversy.[38] Concerned with provider reaction, the carriers would prefer to avoid creating the acrimonious interface with physicians that tends to accompany rigorous utilization review, and thus hesitate to initiate the significant investment of time and resources required to develop the equivalent of model treatment profiles. It is true also that aggressive claims administrators, like U.S. Administrators, have not had time to accumulate long track records. They should be watched very closely over the next few years and their effects carefully documented.

Within the broad arena of health care cost containment, the use of claims form information as a utilization review tool is emerging as an area of particular interest. Increasingly, larger corporations will look for ways to actively intervene in the health care delivery system to eliminate unnecessary units of service or excessive charges. And the focus will increasingly be on the generation of data describing the specific numbers and types of services that health care providers deliver to employees and their dependents. We cannot know at this point whether this approach will work, or whether the tension and professional issues raised as a result of the attempts to constrain practice patterns will cause intolerable provider hostility or revolt. But it is certain that the corporate quest for health data will continue and intensify, and that the data will be analyzed and used in ways that were unimagined a few years ago.

NOTES

1. Executive Office of the President, Council on Wage and Price Stability, *The Complex Puzzle of Rising Health Care Costs: Can the Private Sector Fit it Together?* (Washington, D.C.: U.S.G.P.O. no. 053-003-00255-8, December 1976), hereafter cited as COWPS.

2. COWPS, pp. 131, 135.

3. COWPS, p. 155.

4. COWPS, p. 112.

5. COWPS, p. 132.

6. *Employee Benefit Plan Review Research Reports* is a comprehensive looseleaf service covering pensions and profit sharing; health, life, and disability benefits; unions, and ERISA. Included in the health, life, and disability volumes are several sections relevant to the general considerations of funding and administrative alternatives, data and their uses. The service is available through Charles D. Spencer and Associates, Inc., 222 West Adams Street, Chicago, Illinois 60606. Since it is updated frequently, references to it run the risk of obsolescence but the interested reader can find current information on self-insurance of health benefits in section 331.5 of the Reports.

7. Bruce Spencer, *Group Benefits in a Changing Society* (Chicago, Ill.: Charles D. Spencer and Associates, Inc., 1978), hereafter cited as Spencer, *Group Benefits.*

8. *Employee Benefit Plan Review*, published monthly by Charles D. Spencer and Associates, Inc., 222 West Adams Street, Chicago, Illinois 60606, hereafter cited as EBPR.

9. *Business Insurance*, "the national news magazine of loss prevention, risk financing, and employee benefit management," published biweekly by Crain Communications, Inc., 740 Rush Street, Chicago, Illinois 60611.

10. David A. Weeks, ed., *Rethinking Employee Benefits Assumptions* (New York: The Conference Board, 1978); Seymour Lusterman, ed., *Health-Care Issues for Industry* (New York: The Conference Board, 1974).

11. See, for example, O. D. Dickerson, *Health Insurance* (Homewood, Ill.; Richard D. Irwin, Inc., 1968), John Krizay and Andrew Wilson, *The Patient as Consumer: Health Care Financing in the United States* (Lexington, Mass.: Lexington Books, 1974), Avedis Donabedian, *Benefits in Medical Care Programs* (Cambridge, Mass.: Harvard University Press, 1976).

12. *Source Book of Health Insurance Data* 1977–78 (Washington, D.C.: Health Insurance Institute, 1978). The institute is located at 1850 K Street, N.W., Washington, D.C. 20006.

13. Diana Chapman Walsh and Richard H. Egdahl, *Payer, Provider, Consumer: Industry Confronts Health Care Costs*, Springer Series on Industry and Health Care, no. 1 (New York: Springer-Verlag, Inc., 1977), p. 91.

14. *EBPR Research Reports*, p. 331.5.-1, 9-72 Rev.

15. Ibid.

16. For a concise description of the uses and limitations of a 501(c)(9) trust, see Spencer, *Group Benefits*, pp. 300–301.

17. Spencer, *Group Benefits*, pp. 285–286.

18. Michael B. Jones, Partner, New York Office, Hewitt Associates, presentation at Cornell University Health Program for Business Executives, "Strategies for Controlling Medical Care Costs," Ithaca, New York, May 5, 1977.

19. Spencer, *Group Benefits*, p. 287.

20. Ibid., p. 295.

21. COWPS, p. 24.

22. Spencer, *Group Benefits*, p. 285.

23. Ibid., p. 286.

24. *EBPR Research Reports*, 331.5.-7, 7-71.

25. Spencer, *Group Benefits*, p. 302.

26. Ibid., p. 301.

27. For a special report on agents and brokers of commercial insurance, including a directory, see *Business Insurance's* annual agent/broker profiles issue, August 7, 1978.

28. "Borden Saves 14.2% in 1977 Because of Strict Coordination of Benefits Policy," *EBPR Research Reports* 331.3.-7, 4-78.

29. *Payer, Provider, Consumer*, pp. 23–25.

30. Washington Business Group on Health, "A Private Sector Perspective on the Problems of Health Care Costs," a working paper prepared for the Honorable Joseph Califano, Secretary, Department of Health, Education, and Welfare, Washington, D.C., April 1977, p. 10.

31. Ibid., p. 16.

32. Edmund Faltmayer, "Where Doctors Scramble for Patients' Dollars," *Fortune* (November 6, 1978), pp. 114–120.

33. Richard H. Egdahl and Diana Chapman Walsh, eds., *Industry and HMOs: A Natural Alliance*, Springer Series on Industry and Health Care, no. 5 (New York: Springer-Verlag, Inc., 1978).

34. *Labor-Management Group Position Papers on Health Care Costs 1978* (a limited number of copies is available at cost from the Washington Business Group on Health, 605 Pennsylvania Avenue, S.E., Washington, D.C. 20003).

35. David A. Weeks, *National Health Insurance and Benefit Plans* (New York: The Conference Board, 1974), p. 36.

36. See, for example, Institute of Medicine, *Assessing Quality in Health Care: An Evaluation* (Washington, D.C.: IOM Publication 76-04, November 1976).

37. *Payer, Provider, Consumer*, pp. 16–17.

38. James E. Post, *Risk and Response: Management and Social Change in the American Insurance Industry* (Lexington, Mass.: Lexington Books, 1976), p. 103.

PURCHASER PERSPECTIVES: FOUR CORPORATIONS

American Telephone and Telegraph Company

Richard W. Stone, Michael J. Gulotta, and Donald P. Harrington

AT&T, like most large corporations, has become increasingly concerned in the last several years over the cost of health insurance for its employees. The AT&T plans, underwritten by Blue Cross-Blue Shield and other insurance carriers, cover some three million people, including roughly one million employees and retirees, and their dependents. Health insurance now represents some 5 percent of total payroll, or $750 million, compared to only 1.5 percent when the plans were first introduced in the early 1960s. Of that increase, approximately 2 percent represents plan improvements while 1.5 percent represents increased utilization of the benefit. To investigate approaches to controlling the costs of health insurance, a working group has been created at corporate headquarters, including representatives of the medical, actuarial, systems, and finance departments.

Self-insurance was one of many approaches originally given some consideration. AT&T has self-insured its pension program since 1927 and its lump sum death benefit since the mid-1960s, so the group was quite familiar with the concepts, and analytical process involved in identifying the advantages and disadvantages of self-insurance.

Analyzing Self-Insurance

In reaching a decision whether to self-insure or to contract with an outside insurance carrier for medical benefits "self-insurance" needs to be analyzed in four specific areas: risk charges, cash flow elements, claims administration and other carrier charges.

The first consideration relates to what may be termed the assumption of risk by the employer. The concern here covers the volatility of the claim payments relative to some standard measure, such as payroll. Where the volatility is such that a reliable estimate of the claim payments cannot be made in advance of the time period in question, it is prudent for a company to avoid self-insurance and pay a risk premium to an outside carrier. However, in the case of a very large corporate employer for whom a reliable estimate of claim incurrals can be made, one would expect that the risk charge typically made by a carrier could be avoided. Irrespective of the size of the corporate policyholder, however, the insurer will very likely impose some risk charge, albeit a minimal one. Of further importance is the fact that the financial advantage gained by the elimination of the risk charge may be partially or totally offset by additional expenses associated with the cost of actuarial services required in the determination of the estimated claim payments. Taking account only of the risk charge imposed by the carrier, most firms would probably conclude that self-insurance would seem to be an advantageous approach to providing medical care benefits.

The second consideration is financial in nature and involves health insurance reserves and the time value of money. The reserves held by the carrier are for estimated claims already incurred but not yet finally settled. Claims on which health insurance reserves (and specifically medical care insurance reserves) are typically held by insurers fall into the following three categories:

1. claims due and unpaid
2. claims in course of settlement
3. claims incurred but not reported

The question whether self-insurance is advantageous with regard to these financial considerations is ultimately resolved in terms of the cost of capital to the employer. Can the employer earn more money on these reserves than he is currently being given credit for in the dividend formula, or elsewhere, by the insurance carrier? The elements that enter into the answer relate to the timing of, and arrangements for payment of premiums as well as the amount, if any, of interest credited on reserves held by the insurer. Various mechanisms have been devised by insurers, the effect of which are to compensate at least partially for the time value of money forfeited owing to inability to utilize funds held as health insurance reserves. Among these mechanisms are extended grace periods for the payment of premiums as well as retrospective premium riders (sometimes called facility of payment provisions). Where such mechanisms exist, they reduce the advantage to be gained by self-insuring.

The third consideration relates to the claims administration process. The elements that enter into the claims payment procedure that prove valuable to a corporation relate to third party settlement of disputed claims, analysis of fees in various locations, and in place electronic data processing mechanisms and procedures. From the viewpoint of the large corporate employer, the most valuable service provided by the current arrangement, in light of concern for individual privacy, is the interface between the employer and employee with regard to grievances that naturally arise in the course of claim settlements. Without this interface, employee relations may suffer due to certain denials of claim payment.

The fourth consideration is the element of expense which can be deemed to be peculiar to the insurance industry. Obviously, the foremost element here is the premium tax, which employers have gone to great lengths to avoid through various types of contracts, such as minimum premium, stop loss insurance, or a completely self-insured arrangement. Another item of insurance expense is the charge reflecting the social welfare of the population in general, borne, in part, by the insurance industry and passed on to policyholders. These taxes and charges can be avoided temporarily, but for the longer term, these funds will ultimately have to be provided by the productive segments of the economy. It can thus be argued that the apparent savings generated by self-insurance are not real because these societal expenses will eventually be recovered in an alternative manner.

There is yet another point which should be taken into consideration by employers who contract for hospital and surgical-medical benefits with Blue Cross and Blue Shield plans across the country. Reimbursement mechanisms negotiated with hospitals by Blue Cross plans, for example, enable the hospitals to "give Blue Cross a break," and the insurance saving is passed on to the group policyholder by Blue Cross. There are a number of variables, however, in analyzing the magnitude of the savings generated by contracting with Blue Cross as opposed to an insurance company. The analysis of the financial advantage of insuring with Blue Cross from this point of view is an important factor in the self-insurance equation.

The net result of this analysis for AT&T is that while some short-term savings might be possible through self-insurance, they do not justify implementing it at this time. The basic problem with self-insurance for a large, highly dispersed company like AT&T is that it addresses only the cost of providing the insurance service, and not the much larger cost of the benefits themselves. The decision at AT&T has been to focus on this latter category.

The first step in dealing with the cost of the health benefit is to understand what is now occurring, which means collecting extensive data. Working with Blue Cross, AT&T has decided to create a central data bank which will include information on covered hospital services received by AT&T employees,

HOSPITAL UTILIZATION DATA ELEMENTS

1. Employee/Dependent Status
2. Patients Sex
3. Patients Date of Birth
4. Group Policy Number
5. Hospital I.D. Code
6. Type of Institution
7. Hospital Zip Code
8. Blue Cross Claim Number
9. Date of Admission or Service
10. Date of Discharge
11. Release Code
12. Primary Diagnosis Code
13. Multiple Diagnosis
14. Surgery Indicator
15. Date Surgery Performed
16. Number of Days of Confinement
17. Room and Board Charges
18. Covered Charges
19. Hospital Extras Charges
20. Hospital Extras Covered Charges
21. Amount of Claim Payment
22. Date of Claim Payment
23. Type of Treatment (Outpatient)
24. Multiple Treatment Indicator
25. Total Hospital Charges
26. Total Covered Charges
27. Place of Treatment
28. Blue Cross Plan Code
29. Disposition Code
30. Type of Claim Indicator

retirees, and dependents. The kind of information that will be collected is illustrated in the box. Having a uniform data collection system will serve two main functions. One, AT&T will know to a much greater extent than ever before how it is spending its health care dollar. Two, AT&T will be able to measure the effects of any direct intervention in the health care delivery system. For example, AT&T will be able to explore the effects of the various approaches to administration used by the 69 Blue Cross plans around the country. The hospital utilization monitoring system (HUMS) commenced operations in early 1979. It will operate under the guidelines recommended by the Privacy Protection Study Commission[1] for the confidential management of information collected for research and statistical studies. It should provide the basis for AT&T's long-term efforts to continue to assure high-quality health care as well as to help in the containment of costs.

NOTES

1. Privacy Protection Study Commission, Personal Privacy in an Information Society (United States Government Printing Office/Stock No. 052-003-00395-3, July 1977), chapter 19.

Mobil Oil Corporation

Robert B. Peters, Jack H. Bleuler, and
David H. Winkworth

Rising health care costs have precipitated a clamor for government intervention in the system, particularly for national health insurance (NHI). United States health spending currently exceeds $160 billion annually and is increasing by 15 percent every year. In five years it will double. The private sector has an enormous stake in the problem: of the current $160 billion figure, we expend about $100 billion. It is evident that we in the private sector should be thinking and doing something about this now. We do not believe that the search for a solution should be left to the government and NHI legislation.

At Mobil Oil our current medical plan costs exceed $24 million annually. Since 1965, the total average cost of our Comprehensive Medical Plan for family coverage has grown from $18.20 per month to about $70—a fourfold increase. Factors influencing this rise in plan costs were inflation, increase in plan utilization, plan improvements, and the influence of the malpractice issue on providers.

The first health initiatives by President Carter focused on costs because long-term reform cannot be accomplished unless the problems of runaway costs are brought under control. The president's approach also emphasized the crucial role of the private sector. In his message to Congress concerning the proposed Hospital Cost Containment Act, it was noted for the first time that the cost containment effort: "relied heavily on the initiatives of the private sector. For it to succeed, businesses, unions and insurers, working with providers, must *continue* to pursue innovative techniques for reducing the cost of high quality health care," and "the private sector's response to the challenges of cost containment will help decide its future role in our health care system."

Although the Carter bill appears to be dead, the issue of hospital costs—which represent about 40 percent of total health care expenditures—is very much alive. Congressman Rostenkowski has substituted a bill that places the inpatient care revenues limitation of 9 percent on a stand-by basis. Generally, industry opposes legislation placing a "cap" on revenues because of the price control nature of these approaches. In our opinion, almost any effort to contain health care costs depends on developing innovative strategies involving all the actors in the health care system: company, employee, provider/carrier, and government. What follows are some strategies that we at Mobil Oil believe have potential merit and many of which we are using as the basis for developing our own approach to health care cost control.

Company Innovations to Control Costs

Company innovations fall into the major areas of plan design, plan administration and control, employee communications and health education, and health planning. Mobil Oil, with the help of employees and unions, has introduced many of the following strategies.

Some cost containment features that can be built into the design of the health benefits plan are: deductibles for hospital confinement (for example, $25) and extended benefits (for example, $50–200/per person/per year); coinsurance for surgical benefits and extended benefits (for example, 80 percent plan, 20 percent employee); a coordination of benefits provision, and, if possible, the requirement of employee contributions to the cost of the plan.

Other alterations of the design of the company medical plan can serve to encourage preventive and ambulatory health care, which not only help contain costs but are substantial plan improvements in themselves. For example, Mobil Oil last year added the following cost containment features to its plan:

- Second surgical opinion (Pay 100% vs. 80%)
- Ambulatory surgical care (Pay 100% vs. 80%)
- Extended care facilities (Pay 100% vs. 0)
- Home health care agencies (Pay 100% vs. 80%)
- Outpatient testing (Emphasize 100% pay; add independent laboratory)
- Alcoholism and drug abuse rehabilitation facilities (Pay 100% vs. 0)

Finally, plan designers concerned with cost control can consider a "contribution bonus." In 1977 Mobil Oil announced a bonus, which is the difference, if any, between the maximum company contribution and the total cost of plan coverage (up to the maximum company contribution), to be paid in cash to employees at year end. This bonus, which came to an average of about $55 per family last year, will, we hope, provide an incentive to employees to hold down medical costs.

In the area of plan administration and control, some promising strategies are to combine coverage under a single plan and to provide for experience rating of units so that costs can be more equitably allocated. The administrative costs of handling claims can be reduced by installing a computerized claims-processing system. Also, savings can be realized by becoming self-insured under section 501(c)(9) of the Internal Revenue Code. And finally, a company might wish to consider a cost-effective claims-monitoring and review program.

A company strategy that might lead to significant health care cost savings in the long run is to attempt to improve employee health status and thus reduce the need for many costly services. For instance, a company might consider developing employee communications and education programs aimed at changing health-related life-styles (nutrition, smoking, exercising, use of seat belts, and so on). Some companies are also taking the approach of providing preventive physicals and in-house physical fitness facilities.

In line with our belief that cost control should be a cooperative effort, we feel that a company should become actively involved in community health planning (through participation on local hospital boards and health systems agencies) to help bring health needs and health resources into a better balance. A company might also become actively involved in promoting private sector interests in the shaping of proposed legislation through, for example, serving on committees with groups such as Association of Private Pension and Welfare Plans, the Washington Business Group on Health, the Department of Health, Education, and Welfare, and so on.

Employee (and Dependent) Incentives

Most of the above innovations are designed to encourage the employee to be more realistic in using the medical plan. For example, when medically feasible, employees should have medical treatment done on an outpatient basis in order to avoid the more expensive and less convenient stays in the hospital.

An effective communications program is important to the success of cost control efforts. The program should particularly emphasize advantages to the employee: avoid surgery that is proved unnecessary, avoid overnight stays in a hospital unless necessary, spend more time at home, reduce employee cost because of lower plan costs, and so forth. Also, efforts can be made to enlist the help of dependents in holding down health care costs by sending announcements and other communications to the home. Telling the story effectively is essential to assure that the innovations are understood by employees and their dependents and to enlist their support in efforts to contain rising medical costs.

Provider/Carrier Activities to Contain Costs and Improve Quality

Providers and carriers are the source of many promising cost control strategies, which companies should encourage and support. For instance, health maintenance organizations (HMOs), which emphasize preventive and ambulatory health care, are proving to be cost effective and are having a competitive impact on the traditional fee-for-service health care system. Mobil Oil has been contacted by twenty-five federal/state qualified HMOs, of which eleven have been implemented.

Many hospitals are developing cost containment programs, often implemented with the assistance of the Hospital Self-Assessment Tool (HSAT). Also, hospitals are joining with employers, public officials, and others in voluntary areawide health planning efforts designed to improve the management of community health resources.

Insurance carriers, another crucial component of the health care system, are actively working with companies, industry groups, unions, hospital associations, and others on cost containment matters. They are expanding their health benefit plans to pay for cost-effective types of care both in and out of the hospital; shifting toward the concept of prospective reimbursement of hospitals on the basis of predetermined budgets and rates; and in some cases investing in outpatient care centers, such as HMOs, as alternatives to hospital treatment. Carriers are also undertaking careful claims review programs to make sure that treatment is proper and fees and charges are reasonable in relation to services.

Government Actions

Congress has passed several laws to help control the costs as well as improve the quality of health care services. One of these is a health planning law to end the building of unneeded hospital beds (some reports show over 150,000 excess beds) and the possible duplication of other costly equipment and facilities. Another is a law to assist in the development of HMOs, amended in 1976 and 1978 to further encourage development. Congress has also mandated the setting up of medical review groups called professional standards review organizations (PSROs) throughout the nation in an attempt to make certain that patients covered under Medicare and Medicaid obtain services that are necessary, proper, and of good quality. In addition, a health manpower law has been passed to improve the supply of doctors in underserved areas. And finally, Congress has enacted a consumer health information law to encourage more preventive care and health education of the public.

At the state level, some states now require hospitals to justify their budgets in advance (prospective budget review). States (and others) could also make a contribution by studying long-term reforms needed to control the cost of malpractice insurance.

Summary

Health care cost control is a huge and complicated problem and it is going to take many years for most of our efforts to have any impact. There are not going to be any "quick fixes," but we have to continue searching for solutions. We are hopeful that the concerted efforts of those of us in the private sector—companies, employees, unions, providers, and carriers—will result in viable strategies that should, in the long run, control costs and reduce the pressure on the government to respond with sweeping NHI legislation.

Deere and Company

Kevin Stokeld

Deere and Company has been self-insuring and self-administering its employee health benefits for the past eight years. For a number of reasons, Deere has perhaps more opportunity to control health care costs than many employers. First, we have a large number of United States employees and retirees, currently totalling 56,000; with dependents, the covered group totals some 150,000 people. Second, our covered population is concentrated in small geographic areas—about 80 percent of them live in four locations—which gives us visibility and influence in our discussions with providers. Third, unlike many large corporations, Deere offers one consistent profile of benefits to all beneficiaries, a fact that greatly facilitates our claims management efforts. Finally, Deere owns an insurance company subsidiary.

The decision to go "self-insured" did not rest solely on the perceived advantages of processing our own claims. Avoidance of premium taxes and the

(Extract from a taped interview)

maintaining of reserves on our own books and of course the interest accruing thereon were considered to be the main reasons for "self-insuring." It is possible that if these advantages had not been present we might not have opted to process our own claims.

However, to obtain these fiscal advantages we either had to process claims ourselves or have an independent third party handle them for us. We decided that there was at that time more reason for us to process our own claims than have them handled by a third party.

We began to consider self-insurance back in 1970, when Deere's health insurance premiums (excluding weekly indemnity) were about $18 million a year (no employee contribution). At the time, we were probably doing pretty much what most other large corporations were doing about health insurance; that is we would visit the carrier's home office once a year and in a rather perfunctory manner review the past year's experience. Essentially we were looking at bottom line data without any meaningful analysis. The carrier would propose an increase for the coming year based on a cost-plus formula. There was little sense of urgency in those days to provide detailed data which would allow for health care cost and utilization analysis. Insureds weren't demanding it and carriers weren't providing it. However, in our own case the figures were becoming sufficiently large to point out the need for more and better information.

Although the primary reasons for leaving the carrier to go "self-insured" were to obtain the fiscal advantages already discussed, there were other practical reasons which suggested that we should process our own claims. For one thing we believed that a more coordinated claims management would result from centralizing the claims function as opposed to the carrier's decentralized operation whereby our claims were handled out of as many as twenty claims offices. Also, we could avoid those indirect or overhead charges which most carriers charge to their clients. Finally we believed that we had a more direct interest in working with local health care providers on health care problems than the claims office of a large insurance company headquartered many miles away. For these reasons we decided to handle our own claims effective January 1, 1971.

In 1978 our health care costs will approximate $70 million and the savings which have accrued to the company since 1971 via the avoidance of premium taxes and the interest credits on reserves have in themselves been very significant and have proven the decision to go "self-insurance" to have been correct.

We believe, also, that the decision to process claims ourselves on a centralized basis has also proven to be correct. Not only are claims paid in a consistent and timely manner but the closer scrutiny resulting from our efforts has led to a much tighter application of the coordination of benefits provisions. Currently we handle in excess of 18,000 claims papers each week for just about every conceivable benefit including a full dental and vision program. Furthermore we act as fiscal intermediary for our Medicare retirees. Total administration costs have never exceeded 3 percent of claims paid.

Although we believe that our efforts in claims processing were rewarded, our success was limited in that there were many problems in the so-called health care delivery system which caused costs to escalate and these problems were quite beyond our control. We're referring to the inability of most insurers to cope with the problems of excess utilization especially in the hospital.

As a result we needed to devise a strategy whereby we at Deere could intervene more directly in the health care distribution system. To do this we had one of our managers undertake a special assignment to study Deere's involvement with health care and recommend how the company should proceed. The finished report emphasized the need to do something by preparing a health care cost projection which indicated that if health care costs continued on the same trend as they had for the last five years the company would spend in excess of $2 billion over the next 10-year period. It was recommended that given a total management committment all health care related functions in the company should be brought under one department. Cost containment activities were to be the responsibility of two newly established functions, health care planning and health care services.

As a result the health care department was established effective September 1977, headed up by the director of health care reporting to the vice president of personnel and industrial relations. To insure constant visibility of health care matters the director of health care and the manager of health care planning are members of a special executive committee which also includes two corporate senior vice presidents and one vice president plus the medical director. This committee constitutes possibly the most important change in our organization giving, as it does, immediate and continuous access to top management. If direct intervention in the health care distribution system is to be successful such access is imperative.

Direct Intervention in the Health Care System

Although cost containment has been discussed for many years it is only recently coming into its own mainly for the reason that costs are now recognized to be unnecessarily high. Historically, the cost containment function was considered to be an adjunct of the claims department. Cost containment activities were normally limited to denying or reducing claim payments and never really were able to get at the basic problems of overutilization.

As a result we made a basic distinction between the production aspects of claims processing and the function of cost containment. Aside from ensuring that all appropriate in-house audit techniques were in place the claims processing unit would function essentially as a production unit. It would work according to the processing manual which would be prepared jointly by cost containment and claims processing personnel.

On the other hand the cost containment function acts as the company's spokesman in all health care activities not associated with the processing of claim papers. This covers provider relations (hospitals, physicians, dentists, pharmacists), PSRO activities, medical society and foundation relationships and local HSAs. In addition the manager of health care services is responsible for ensuring that employees act as hospital board members where appropriate and that they are continuously kept informed of the company's involvements and interests in local hospital problems.

In establishing the new health care department we recognized the importance of providing a system which could provide meaningful health cost data for the cost containment function. A position was created to assume this all important function. As a result a much improved computer data system is now being developed for our claims processors (on line using ICDA 9 CM and CPT (4) coding). This data function works hand in hand with the cost containment function and ensures the data requested is in the format requested and as a result can be used for cost containment purposes.

Finally and perhaps of greatest significance we have been very active in the last twelve months in promoting the formation of an HMO in the Quad Cities. We believe that the open panel model has much greater potential for us in that it is less disruptive to the medical communities and the probable number of enrollees will far exceed what we might expect under the closed panel approach.

Deere's self-assumed role is to act as a catalyst in bringing together the interested parties, that is, the providers and the purchasers of health care. Naturally the issue is a very sensitive one and Deere has been careful to keep the doctors constantly informed of our interests in this area. Since February 1978 we have been meeting with representatives of the local medical societies and in September we proposed that an IPA-HMO would be in the best interests of the community. We are currently visiting a number of IPAs with the representatives of the medical society and hope to have an official response to our proposal from the physicians by the end of the year.

Polaroid Corporation

Galt Grant

Polaroid Corporation is a nonunionized employer with approximately 14,000 of its 15,000 domestic United States employees working in plants located throughout the eastern part of Massachusetts. The company manufactures instant cameras, film, and light-polarizing products. During the 1970s, Polaroid underwent a substantial change in operations: it took over camera assembly operations from its former supplier, added facilities to manufacture SX-70 film, and built a negative manufacturing facility. Over this period, the company increased its domestic employee population by approximately 50 percent, particularly through the camera assembly operation, which requires a large number of assembly line workers.

Polaroid's employee benefits, such as retirement, disability, death, and medical benefits, are administered through a Benefits Committee consisting of five corporate officers who act as plan administrator and fiduciary for purposes of the Employee Retirement Income Security Act. A Plan Manager Committee, made up of representatives from the Personnel and Finance divisions, is responsible for the day-to-day administration of the benefit program.

Health Benefits Package

Employee health benefits include Blue Cross-Blue Shield Master Medical insurance, Medex III insurance supplementing Medicare, the Harvard Community Health Plan (an HMO), and a dental insurance plan. Polaroid also maintains a medical clinic, staffed by company doctors and nurses, which provides care directly to employees for both industrial and nonindustrial injuries and illnesses. Participation in either Blue Cross-Blue Shield or the Harvard Community Health Plan is mandatory unless the employee's spouse has medical insurance elsewhere; the dental insurance plan was elective when initiated but became mandatory for all employees with one year's service hired after April 1, 1977. The company pays 75-80 percent of the cost of each of these insurance programs, emphasizing the belief that employee sharing of the cost leads to greater appreciation of the benefit and to the awareness that employees have a stake in higher (or lower) medical costs.

The Blue Cross-Blue Shield Master Medical program reimburses inpatient hospital and doctor bills in full and, after a $25 per person (or $50 per family) deductible every six months, 80 percent of routine office visits and most outpatient services. Average enrollment in 1977 at Polaroid in the Master Medical program totalled 10,400 regular employees, plus 500 retirees and active employees over age 65 enrolled in the Medex program. The cost in 1977 was approximately $10.3 million, of which about $8 million was paid by the company and the remainder by employees.

The Harvard Community Health Plan provides benefits similar to those of Blue Cross-Blue Shield Master Medical except that most services are provided by the HMO's two facilities and coverage is somewhat broader, including physical examinations and other services at a nominal one-dollar per visit charge. The average enrollment is 335 employees—less than 3 percent of regular employees. Almost half of these are individual memberships versus approximately 28 percent individual memberships for Blue Cross-Blue Shield. The cost in 1977 was approximately $300,000.

The Polaroid Dental Program, which provides full coverage for regular checkups and 50-60 percent coverage on dental repair work, had an average enrollment in 1977 of about 8,900 employees. The plan was introduced as of April 1, 1977, and developed a total cost in that year of approximately $1.15 million, of which the company paid 75 percent.

Funding Health Benefits

Polaroid's general philosophy of funding employee benefits is to assume as much risk as economically feasible and to pay its own way, particularly with respect to benefits, like medical insurance, that have a high frequency of claims. Polaroid attempts to obtain maximum use of any reserves that might be necessary in connection with the benefit programs.

The Harvard Community Health Plan does not meet this objective since it is not funded on a loss cost plus expense basis. Instead, rates are calculated on a flat amount per employee and are not directly affected by Polaroid's actual loss experience, except as it relates to the group as a whole.

On the other hand, the Master Medical program is funded through what amounts to an administrative services only approach: Blue Cross-Blue Shield is reimbursed the cost of claims paid on behalf of group members plus a handling charge. This is particularly advantageous to the company and plan members from a cost standpoint because of the arrangements that Blue Cross-Blue Shield has made within the Commonwealth of Massachusetts. First, hospitals accept, on average, a 5 percent discount on claims submitted through Blue Cross. Second, participating physicians accept 95 percent of usual and customary fees as full payment. Blue Shield cannot pay benefits to nonparticipating physicians and physicians cannot bill patients for the remaining 5 percent of usual and customary expenses. Finally, because Blue Cross and Blue Shield are nonprofit organizations, premiums paid to them are not subject to state tax. As a result of these factors, in Massachusetts at least, it is impossible to improve on Blue Cross-Blue Shield's arrangements from the standpoint of administrative and other costs per dollar of actual benefit paid. Also, the plan is popular with employees because the Blue Cross-Blue Shield card is widely accepted, and upon presentation to hospitals and physicians results in no claim forms for the employee to complete for the vast majority of covered services.

Much of the cost-effectiveness of this arrangement disappears outside of Massachusetts under the existing plan because coverage for participating physicians' services is based on usual and customary charges as determined by Blue Shield of Massachusetts. (An exception is California where the arrangement is similar to that in Massachusetts.) If there is a balance for covered services rendered outside of Massachusetts, the plan will pay 80 percent of the difference but the physician can bill the employee for the excess amount.

The dental plan is written through an affiliate of Blue Cross-Blue Shield of Massachusetts, the Massachusetts Dental Service Corporation. The arrangement as respects participating dentists is similar to that of Blue Cross-Blue Shield with doctors, except that at best only about 90 percent of the dentists in the state participate and the Massachusetts Dental Service Corporation is allowed by law to make benefit payments to nonparticipating dentists. The funding arrangement is similar to the Blue Cross-Blue Shield Master Medical program except for certain rate and maximum premium guarantees.

Because of the particular advantage of Blue Cross-Blue Shield's arrangements within the Commonwealth of Massachusetts, formally self-insured medical plans do not have the same appeal to Massachusetts employers that they may have in certain other jurisdictions. In effect, however, Polaroid's arrangement amounts to self-insurance since no premium taxes are paid, cash flow is maximized, and the retention is at a reasonable level.

Cost Containment Efforts

There are several cost containment devices built into the Blue Cross-Blue Shield system in addition to their financial arrangements with the hospitals and doctors. These include peer review and a coordination of benefits provision which has only recently begun to be utilized in Massachusetts to any degree. However, there is no current method by which an employer can assess whether the most cost-effective medical practices are being followed; second opinion procedures may be desirable but are not as yet in widespread use in Massachusetts. In fact, there is little that Polaroid can do independently to control costs, other than to provide free physical examinations and employee health care at its in-house clinic and to cooperate with its insurance carriers and with any provider organization in trying to cut back overutilization of health care. One alternative, cutting back on benefits, simply is not feasible or desirable.

HMOs are often seen as a possible means of cost control, but as evidenced by the less than 3 percent enrollment, the Harvard Community Health Plan has not proven to be an attractive alternative for many Polaroid employees. Part of the reason for this could be that the plan's two facilities are not easily accessible to most employees, who work at plants in a number of eastern Massachusetts locations.

From a company point of view, one should note that Harvard Community Health Plan rates have increased faster in the past four years than have those of Polaroid's Master Medical Program, and actual Harvard Community Health Plan costs are now higher than those being paid for the Master Medical Program. Also, under current HMO funding arrangements it is not possible to purchase benefits on a group basis. A company therefore has to pay full administrative costs and the doctors get the advantages of cash flow; the result is that HMO costs (in Polaroid's experience at least) have not been less than Master Medical insurance. It is possible, however, that the emphasis on preventive health care under the HMO concept may have longer range cost advantages.

Conclusion

The decision whether to self-insure medical benefits must take into consideration the overall financial condition and funding philosophy of a corporation. The company must measure the level of risk versus the amount of company money an insurance company requires to assume that risk, as well as assess relative cash flow and administrative charges of an insured versus a self-insured arrangement. Regardless of whether a particular corporation is insured or self-insured, its long-term premium, if the company is of any size, will be based on its actual loss experience. But retention of reserves, reduction of premium tax, and lowering of administrative expenses can result in real savings, and it is incumbent upon a company to investigate such methods of cost control. Obviously, self-insurance in and of itself can only seek the most effective financial manner of minimizing costs; it does not address cost control of health care itself.

ADMINISTERING THE BENEFIT: THIRD-PARTY VIEWS

Prudential Insurance Company of America

Lesley L. Ralson

There can be little doubt that the assumption of some insurance risk by the large employer is an appropriate method of financing employee health benefits, and the marketplace has responded by offering a wide variety of such arrangements. This phenomenon is generally described as the movement toward self-insured plans or, more correctly, uninsured plans.

The insurance industry cannot be surprised at this development. Uninsured health benefit plans are the natural culmination of trends that have been at work for many years within our industry. In fact, the motivations that are now leading employers toward uninsured plans have their beginnings in what was the commercial insurance industry's first major innovation in the employee benefits field—experience rating.

The Roots of "Self-Insurance"

Fifteen years ago, most employee benefit plans were fully insured and experience-rated. Premiums were set annually in advance at a level intended to cover expected cash claims, with some margin for fluctuation, necessary reserves, and the insurance company's retention which included expenses and risk-sharing charges. The employer's selection of a carrier was determined primarily on the basis of the lowest retention, with minimal regard to the quality or even the amount of service the carrier was to provide. There was certainly no discussion of cost containment, because it could be construed as an attempt to avoid paying legitimate claims. Most employers wanted some flexibility in determining which claims would be paid and often insisted that certain ineligible claims be paid—especially for management employees. Failure to pay such claims could result in transfer of the coverage to a more cooperative insurance company.

Many employers began to realize that if they stayed with the same carrier, they would eventually carry the full risk of their plan because the rerate procedures would recoup any deficits incurred in a given year. In an effort to help the employer postpone the impact of rerates necessitated by the inflationary spiral in health care costs, the insurance companies started offering retrospective rating. Under this arrangement, premiums paid during the year were only an estimate of the costs; the final premium was determined at the end of the year.

Since most of these retrospective agreements had some upper limit, or "cap," on the employer's liability, the risk for the insurance company remained the same. If claims should exceed the cap, any deficits could be recovered in future years, as long as the employer stayed with the same carrier. If this concept is carried to an extreme, a retrospective rating arrangement becomes much like a minimum premium plan (MPP). Under MPP, the employer self-insured most benefits and the insurance company assumed a layer of coverage on top of the base risk. In a typical plan, the insurance premium was about 10 percent of the total cost of the plan. Since the other 90 percent was not insured, the plan escaped state premium taxes which average about 2 percent but are as high as 4 percent in some states.

The tight money situation of the early 1970s led to pressure for the assumption of another function by the employer—holding the unrevealed claims reserve, which often amounted to 30-40 percent of a year's premium. Many employers felt that such a large amount of cash was better invested in their company than accumulating at the relatively lower after tax portfolio rates that carriers were able to offer. Group insurance carriers sought additional ways to accommodate large employers' cash flow through such devices as deferred premiums and extended grace periods.

By this time, most of the elements of an "insuring" relationship were no longer part of the large employer's health benefits plan. Employers did, however, remain interested in purchasing such insurance company services as claims processing, actuarial advice, and communications to employees. Thus, there arose a market for the administrative services only (ASO) contract. Another spur to growth of ASO arrangements in the last few years was the enactment of the Employee Retirement Income Security Act of 1974 (ERISA). Many employers interpret ERISA as preempting state regulation, thereby making ASO a vehicle for escaping state-mandated health insurance benefits as well as state premium taxes.

What Insurers Can Offer

Prudential's approach to the market derives from an analysis of what going uninsured can do for the employer and what it cannot do. For groups that are large enough to assume the risk we offer ASO and MPP contracts. This posture has actually proven difficult to maintain in the marketplace, because other carriers, consultants, and administrators are marketing ASO arrangements to groups whose volume is a fraction of what we think a reasonable spread of risk should be. Properly conceived, these arrangements can be economical to the extent that they improve cash flow and escape certain regulatory or tax burdens.

However, they do not help to contain health care costs because they do not alter the health care delivery system. Liability under a given plan of health benefits covering a given group will not be reduced by simply transferring the risk or the payment function, because the health care needs of the group, the structure of the system providing for those needs, and, consequently, the cost of health benefits will not change as a result of such a transfer. It could be argued that going uninsured increases the employer's motivation to be concerned with the cost effectiveness of health care providers, since the effects of increases or reductions in cost will be felt more immediately and directly, but I have no evidence that uninsured employers get better performance from the health care delivery system.

On balance, self-insured approaches do have some advantages for employers who are large enough to make the assumption of risk reasonable. The most important decision for such an employer is who will pay the claims—his own organization, an insurance carrier, or some other third party? There are compelling reasons why full administration by an insurance carrier under an MPP or ASO arrangement is desirable. Many of these reasons relate to resources that an insurance carrier has for legitimately reducing claims costs which employers could duplicate only at very substantial cost, if at all:

> A carrier such as Prudential has efficient, sophisticated on-line teleprocessing computer claim payment systems that enable claim examiners, wherever located, to have instant access to important data such as employee eligibility, prior claim history, provider information, and reasonable and customary fees. These systems minimize mathematical errors, provide screens that enable the examiner to spot potential fraud and/or abuse situations, and serve to monitor the accuracy and consistency of claim payments.

> We can provide claim analysis programs that enable us and/or our clients to isolate and address factors that contribute to poor overall claim experience. These programs are used to monitor dental, hospital, surgical,

and/or disability claim experience and offer many analytical variables that can isolate experience by hospital, doctor/dentist, diagnosis or procedure, age, sex, plant location, and so forth.

With many households containing two or more working people and with many people holding more than one job, it is not uncommon for a household to be covered under more than one employee benefits program. Most group insurance plans, insured or uninsured, have a coordination of benefits (COB) provision that limits total payment to an insured with multiple group coverage to no more than 100 percent of eligible expenses. Good COB administration requires experience in identifying multiple coverage situations and in dealing with other carriers. If well performed, COB can result in benefit dollar savings—sometimes as high as 10 percent of the claim cost.

Many plans today cover all or part of "reasonable and customary" charges for dental, medical, and/or surgical services. While there is controversy regarding the use of this device for purposes of cost containment, Prudential has been a leader in developing "profile" systems that enable us to implement it effectively and efficiently. We take the fee information routinely captured by our automated claim payment systems and array it to reflect the past twelve months' experience, by procedure and provider, in 244 areas of the country. The results are then fed back into our claim payment systems so that our examiners have instant access to the appropriate charge level for a given procedure no matter where service was provided. However, since physicians' charges represent less than one-third of total insured medical expense and the majority of charges do fall within the reasonable and customary guidelines, the actual savings from this program are not very large.

Prudential, through its own efforts and those of the Health Insurance Association of America to which we belong, aggressively pursues and utilizes all available prompt payment hospital discount programs. These programs can reduce charges for hospital claims by 2–5 percent. Moreover, Prudential has an equally aggressive policy of auditing hospital claims involving high dollar amounts, long confinement, or abnormal relationships between ancillary and room and board charges. These activities are often very effective in reducing charges on an individual claim as well as indicating to the hospital that we review bills and will seek adjustments where appropriate.

Prudential has been among the leaders in establishing innovative cost containment programs such as second opinion for elective surgery. While such programs have not yet gained wide acceptance or been fully utilized, they can, when properly installed, produce savings. As is the case with many new programs, effectiveness and utilization will grow with maturity and exposure. We have the expertise and experience to establish and run such programs for our clients.

In addition to the actual processing of claims, proper administration of any health benefits program requires extensive legal and medical consultation by specialists experienced in health care financing issues. A large carrier has far greater resources than it would be feasible for a single employer to maintain. The potential legal liabilities that the administrator of a health benefits plan must assume are enormous. They may include defending disputed claim payments, liability in the event of error, and the claim fiduciary responsibility under ERISA.

Prudential acts in these capacities for insured plans. It is part of our purpose and we feel quite comfortable assuming such a responsibility. We can also perform similar functions for uninsured plans that we administer.

Another factor that argues for insurance carrier administration is the trend toward dual and multiple choice arrangements for health benefits. As the market share of HMOs increases, the size of both insured and uninsured groups will diminish. In some companies as many as 50 percent of the employees have already chosen the HMO option. Some employers could find in the future that, having established the systems and personnel for self-administration, the covered group has decreased in size to the point where self-administration is cost ineffective. Most employers should consider high participation in HMOs a desirable thing, since HMOs have a genuine potential for achieving cost containment in the way it has to be achieved—by reforming the organization and delivery of health care services. These savings can amount to as much as $100 annually for each employee enrolled in an HMO, and in many cases they accrue directly to the employer. It does not make sense, therefore, for an employer to set himself at cross-purposes by investing in systems whose effectiveness could be eliminated by a successful HMO enrollment.

In summary, we believe that economics and the marketplace have spoken clearly on the role of uninsured plans—they are "right" for many large employers. At the same time, they are a natural extension of the kinds of relationships group insurance carriers have developed with their clients over a period of many years. There is no substitute for the involvement of a first-rate, experienced carrier in the day-to-day administration of an MPP or ASO plan.

Blue Cross-Blue Shield of Greater New York

Steven Sieverts

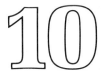

Some authorities are speaking out in favor of self-insurance of health benefits for organizations that are large enough to predict their risk with reasonable accuracy. Their cases generally focus on allegedly greater management control over losses, lower administrative costs, and maximized fiscal returns on cash flow. At least five arguments can be advanced, however, as to why self-insurance is probably inappropriate and self-defeating in most circumstances.

What follows is a case for health insurance by carriers rather than by employers and unions. I submit that self-insurance fails to fill the bill with respect to cost containment and quality assurance; the present and future role of government; consumer protection; the privacy of medical records; and the potential for change and innovation. I will not address the issues of comparative administrative costs and money management returns, except to note that the marketplace will tend to pick the winners in the competition in this arena—and to note further that even very minor shifts in health care expenditure patterns tend to dwarf large shifts in the administrative expenses of health insurance. It can often cost dollars in benefit payments to save pennies in overhead.

Self-Insurance Cannot Do Much for Cost Containment and Quality Assurance

Health care costs and quality are variable in virtually infinite ways. Most medical care decisions—80 percent or more in some authorities' evaluations— are physician-generated. Physicians' choices are heavily influenced by the range of available resources, by the patterns of local medical practice, and by rules and standards of the hospitals where they practice. Hence, cost control efforts must have provider behavior as a prime target; the decisions as to kinds of services to offer and utilize; the choices as to efficacy, efficiency, and productivity; and the choices as to price, are the key factors to influence. They have as great or greater impact on cost levels than do the unpredictable happenstances of illness and injury. The crucial question is the role that the group purchaser can play in altering those factors.

One way in which the purchaser can exert pressure on hospitals and physicians is to deny payment of claims if they represent unnecessary or inappropriate care. This is a very limited tool, but there is some evidence that providers do tend to accommodate their patterns of service to meet the insurers' patterns of coverage. Whether the selective denial of claims is consistently an effective cost containment or quality assurance device is doubtful, however, especially if a net consequence is a shift of care from inexpensive non-covered service to costly covered service. In any event, the denial of claims is a difficult process that distresses both the unpaid provider and (except in "hold harmless" environments) the uncovered consumer.

A second and much more important purchaser influence on providers is the kind that is brought to bear *before* care is rendered. Hospitals can be motivated to take steps to become more efficient without compromising quality. They can make development decisions that support cost-saving (and clinically stronger) regionalized services. They can institute scheduling systems to reduce length-of-stay. Standards can be promulgated and made influential in such matters as the appropriateness of marginally useful diagnostic studies, surgical procedures, and the like. Alternative services with enhanced cost-effectiveness can be developed, such as ambulatory surgery programs, home health programs, and pre-admission diagnostic programs. Quantum improvements in institutional effectiveness can be achieved with modern technology such as automated medical information systems.

Various constructive pressures can be brought to bear on hospitals and physicians in these matters. Group purchasing power can be used creatively, not in the sense of hard-headed market coercion which would surely generate substantial community backlash, but rather in the form of multiple programs to improve utilization patterns and medical care efficacy, to promote efficient hospital management, and to reshape and shrink the health care delivery system along more cost-effective lines.

What does it take to foster such programs? First and foremost, it requires *scale*. If a payer covers only one or even three or six out of every hundred people in a community, it probably lacks the "clout" with providers necessary to stimulate constructive change. But suppose that the payer either singly or through cooperative effort is involved with 20 percent, 30 percent, or 40 percent of a population. Then substantial programs, for example to provide diagnostic studies on an outpatient basis prior to hospitalization, can be effectively developed with a reasonable expectation that the providers will adapt. With scale, a program can offer positive incentives to hospitals that conform to specified objectives, such as by showing that their medical care evaluation programs are having demonstrable impact, or by showing substantial gains in energy conservation.

The second requirement for a payer to develop effective programs is *capability*. Experience has shown that unless substantial administrative and medical know-how is applied to the task, efforts to induce change are usually futile and often expensively counterproductive. For example, working with hospitals to establish ambulatory surgery as a substitute for hospitalization requires the capability to develop protocols and to monitor performance, to assure that the ambulatory surgery is not primarily a nonefficacious and costly transfer of minor procedures from physicians' offices and hospital emergency departments. A more pervasive example of the need for professional capability is in the analysis of medical care utilization to implement active intervention with hospitals and physicians whose practices seem to reflect inappropriate patterns. In the hands of the inexpert, this can range from wasted effort to induced counterreactions from providers who resent having to cope with what they perceived to be incompetent bureaucrats.

Third, effective programs require *data*. One must have an extensive data base in order to analyze existing utilization patterns to propose reasonable directions for change. If one hopes to stimulate hospitals to manage their energy consumption or their personnel scheduling or their commodities purchasing more effectively, one must have the data upon which to build such initiatives.

Finally, effective efforts at change require a *mandate*: there must be solid evidence that the payer represents substantial interests. A major reason, after all, why cost and quality control programs have not burgeoned in the past is that hardly any significant forces were demanding action. Until the 1970s, only a few state governments and many Blue Cross and Blue Shield plans were calling for change, and challenges to them frequently questioned whether they had any significant social support. After all, for decades the federal government's pressures were mostly for more and better health services and facilities for more people. This apparently reflected a broad social consensus. With the economy booming, and with employers expressing more concern about improving the quality of fringe benefits than about cost trends, cost containment lacked a strong constituency.

What does it take to develop the scale, the capability, the data, and the mandate to have a solid impact on the costs and quality of health care in a community? With the rare exception of the relatively isolated small community in which a single employer dominates the labor market, it would seem to require collective and cooperative effort. In most communities, a single employer or other single entity by itself cannot have much influence on the health care delivery system. What is needed is aggregated action. And what is health insurance if not a kind of collective undertaking by the parties that have to pay for health services? In reality and in potential, the nonprofit health service prepayment plans in many regions are at present the only health insurers that have the scale, the capability, and the data to take direct action to affect local health care delivery systems. Because they share the mandate, however, commercial group insurers could also become more effective levers—particularly through cooperative effort.

A unique feature of the Blue Cross plans is their contractual relationships with institutions. These contracts can and do form the basis for a variety of cost-containing and quality-enhancing measures, including such important tools as controlled reimbursement, institutional audit, telecommunications with hospitals, utilization review, and technical/professional assistance. Similarly, if somewhat less pervasively, Blue Shield plans have developed and implemented multiple ways of dealing with medical costs through their unique contractual arrangments with physicians in many areas. It is striking how few commercial health insurance companies or self-insured programs have any programs of this kind. As a result, this argument against self-insurance and self-administration is also an argument against insured programs, unless those programs, by themselves or through alliances, cover a large enough proportion of the population to support a capable cost containment and quality assurance activity aimed at the providers.

Self-Insurance Will Accelerate Total Governmental Takeover of Health Insurance and Health Care

There are at least three reasons why any large-scale move toward self-insurance and self-administration of health care benefits would speed up the growth of governmental regulation both of the health care delivery system and of health insurance, including self-administered and self-insured programs.

First, the more fragmented the private purchaser/payer sector in health care, the less impact that sector is likely to have on containing the costs of health care, for the reasons described above. And the weaker the marketplace forces in shaping the decisions of the health care providers, the stronger the invitation to governmental interventions. Experience suggests, however, that regardless of how well meant such interventions may be, they usually work poorly in achieving their commendable objectives—and frequently stimulate unintended side effects and large hidden costs.

The issue, therefore, is not whether public regulatory efforts will continue, because they will, both in areas where they are likely to achieve some of their goals, and in areas where history suggests that they are liable to costly bungling. Rather, the issue is whether the marketplace forces represented by private sector purchasers and payers interacting with health care providers can show sufficient effectiveness in cost containment to head off ineffective major public interventions, and to encourage government to make constructive use of voluntary initiatives.

If a large-scale move toward self-insurance takes shape, with the resultant fragmenting of purchasing power into more and more, smaller and smaller action units, the likelihood of significant uses of that power grows dim.

Second, government is rightly interested in guarding consumer interests. The public has come to expect a number of protections from health insurance which self-insured and self-administered programs, however, appear to have difficulty in assuring. For example, employees feel entitled to have their coverages continue uninterrupted if they should leave a particular job, and they expect their coverages to be useful if they incur substantial medical expenses while away from their home regions. Moreover, citizens increasingly are demanding accountability from their health insurers in such matters as promptness in reimbursing the full costs of covered services, and fairness in the definitions of what services are to be covered. In addition, the public expects assurance of coverage should an employer or welfare fund get into financial difficulty. All these protections cost money, whether they are mandated by law or won at the bargaining table. If a self-insured, self-administered plan is able, for a time, to avoid these obligations, it will, for a time, save some costs. But only for a time.

With any substantial growth in insurance and administration of health care benefits by entities not now effectively regulated by insurance laws, legislative intervention becomes inevitable. Not only will self-insured programs be held responsible for maintaining adequate reserves to provide assured protection to covered consumers, but they will also probably be compelled to conform to multiple legal mandates in such matters as providing convenient coverage while away from home and assuring departing employees the right to convert their coverages to self-payment. In time, to phrase it bluntly, governmental regulation seems sure to impose on self-insured and self-administered programs the same obligations it imposes on group health insurance—at what seems sure to become greater cost than when such obligations are assumed by insurers with economies of scale. The current absence of such legal obligations for self-insured plans creates apparent cost savings in the short run, but these are unlikely to endure.

Third, it appears that the debates about the enactment of national health insurance will continue for another several years before Congress enacts and a president signs an NHI law. Much of the dispute is over the extent of the responsibility which non-governmental entities will be able to retain over benefits, benefit administration, risk management, quality assurance, and cost containment. Some of the strongest current voices are urging virtually total federal (or federal/state) administration and control, despite the apparent absence of credible evidence that the public sector in this country can perform any or all of these functions effectively, or that the electorate either wishes or would be aided by nationwide uniformity in these matters.

NHI will be enacted largely because of the valid concern that tens of millions of Americans are currently without anything approaching adequate health insurance coverage. Despite the strength of this imperative, action on NHI continues to be delayed, in part because of the lack of consensus as to whether employers, unions, and other payers for group health coverage should continue to have a meaningful role on behalf of their workers and workers' families. The actual debate frequently focuses on the extent to which insurance companies and data processing firms might contract to perform specific administrative functions under a federally conducted NHI program. This is a secondary issue, of course. The broader question, which is rarely brought up, is whether nongovernmental group purchasers will have any say at all in fashioning the benefits and controlling the costs of the health insurance they pay for—as they do not now have with the Medicare program.

   If a major portion of group health coverage becomes self-insured and self-administered, with the consequent predictable weakening of health insurance's aggregate capability (both real and potential) of affecting cost containment and quality assurance in the health care delivery system, the likelihood of significant nongovernmental forces in implementing NHI becomes more remote. There are already powerful interest groups that are scornful of virtually any private effort to induce socially beneficial changes in health care. They feel free to point at communities or regions in this country in which the health insurance sector seems not to have done much to contain costs effectively, even though there are many more communities and regions in which local prepayment plans (usually in cooperation with government, the hospitals, major employers and unions, and other groups such as professional standards review organizations and areawide health planning agencies) have done extraordinarily well. If these anti-private sector forces can point also to major private purchasers who have chosen no longer to rely on existing non-governmental health insurance plans, they will surely claim that as support for their assertion that only government can control health care costs, and as evidence that only government can be counted on to provide assured protection for consumers.

Self-Insurance Fails to Provide Adequate Protection to Consumers

   A group's decision to self-insure and self-administer its health benefits is, in effect, a judgment that no competitive insurer could run the program as well as the group can itself. There are important services, however, that become exceedingly difficult, if not impossible, for a self-administered group to provide to its beneficiaries at satisfactory levels. It may be that the group can do well in processing and paying ordinary claims for local services to local members, but that is by no means the totality of what consumers expect from health insurance.

   For example, how does a self-administered program provide meaningful protection to a consumer who is traveling or who is living and working in a community remote from the group's offices? The health insurer should be able to give an identification card to employees and dependents that permits admission to any hospital without any need for costly advance deposits or aggravating credit checks. A 24-hour toll-free telephone confirmation system might conceivably substitute for the security of an ID card bearing the logo of Blue Cross-Blue Shield or of a recognized commercial insurer—but at what cost?

A second service that self-insured programs have difficulty in assuring is the conversion, without any loss of continuity, of group coverage to direct-pay coverage when a person leaves the insured group. This has come to be regarded by Americans as a kind of basic health right, and state insurance commissioners are increasingly insisting that group health insurers provide this privilege as a legal obligation. Perhaps this feature could be bought as a separate package from a health insurer, but the costs could be high and the problems of determining liability, particularly the early months after a former employee converts, could be most vexatious.

A third service that the public increasingly expects relates to the uncommon but not rare instances of fraud, abuse, and negligence on the part of the providers, both institutional and professional, especially in those situations in which patients are being exploited or victimized. It takes sophisticated analytic capabilities and a considerable data base to detect and deal with these cases. Medical fraud and abuse are often difficult to prosecute, not only because of the sometimes indistinct line between acceptable practice and unacceptable, but also because the principal evidence is frequently buried in inadequately maintained medical records which themselves are largely prepared by the people under suspicion.

In their dealings with health insurance carriers, large and small groups are coming to expect a capability to discover and deal appropriately with the occasional wayward physician, dentist, podiatrist, hospital, and so on—especially in those situations in which patients are being exploited or victimized. Only the rare self-insured entity would have the capacity to detect any but the most blatant abuses; rarer still would be the professional skills (medical, investigative, and legal), the data base, and the will to prosecute. Absent this capacity, any third-party payer may find itself inadvertently stimulating rather than helping to prevent abuse in health care delivery, just as some Medicaid programs, may have, by their lack of capability and purpose in these matters, unintentionally encouraged exploitative practices and the development of unscrupulous "Medicaid mills" and the like. Clearly the most effective preventive measures are those which are perceived to put the potential malefactor at substantial risk of being discovered and prosecuted. In few areas could a single self-administered health insurance program have sufficient scope to create a "preventive" environment in the community—but it is not difficult to imagine that with growth, a multiplicity of small programs, each with a weak capacity to deal with fraud and abuse, might well stimulate increases in such behavior by the small number of unscrupulous practitioners and professionals.

Self-Insurance Raises Serious Questions About the Privacy of Medical Records

Whoever administers a health insurance program must have full access to the records of the medical care received by beneficiaries. This is particularly so with respect to paying claims for hospitalizations and other kinds of care that represent large cost items.

Hospitals and physicians have both legal and ethical obligations to maintain the privacy of these records. Further, consumers expect that when intimate information is entered into the files maintained on their medical care, they can be sure that only those with a legitimate purpose will be able to obtain access to that information.

It was long ago well established that third-party payers have such a legitimate purpose. In order to establish whether health services are covered, payers obviously have to be able to examine the records of those services. In exercising their functions which require obtaining the medical records of beneficiaries, insurers—universally, one supposes—guard the confidentiality of those records as carefully, if not more carefully, than do the institutions and practitioners who create and maintain them.

No doubt, a self-insured, self-administered health insurance program would also be professional and scrupulous in shielding medical records from scrutiny by outside parties, but the troublesome question is whether the employer should have access to personal information about employees and their families. Is it realistic to expect that an organization will be able to claim credibly that it scrutinizes these records for one purpose—ascertaining fiscal responsibility—without also making use of the data for entirely different corporate purposes? For example, if an employee is under treatment for alcoholism or acute depression or a venereal disease or an abortion, and the employer's administrators have detailed records of those illnesses and treatments, the reasonable observer would presume that the information could be used in ways detrimental to the employees' wishes, if not their legal rights. It may be too much to expect an employer to have knowledge of an employee's heart condition or malignancy, and to entirely ignore that kind of information in making job assignments or promotions.

Leaving aside the issue of potential misuse of medical records information, there are also growing concerns in this country about invasions of privacy *per se*. Where in the past there may have been considerable tolerance of officialdom's intrusions into people's personal spheres, both legislative and judicial law are increasingly reflecting an apparently strong public feeling against such intrusions. (The recent judicial mandate to law enforcement agencies to destroy people's criminal arrest records is an interesting case in point.) Increasingly, neither hospitals nor insurers are willing to release information about individuals' medical care without a valid subpoena.

It seems highly likely that sooner or later, self-insured and self-administered group health insurance programs will be faced with the issue of whether, as representatives of employers and/or unions, they have a legitimate right to intimate information about their members—and their members' families—health conditions and treatments. A disturbing corollary to this is the question of how much needed health care might be avoided by covered persons precisely because they would not want their employers or their colleagues to know about their conditions. This seems especially probable in such areas as drug addiction, alcoholism, and psychiatric problems.

Health insurers can virtually guarantee the privacy of medical records, even while furnishing to the insured groups detailed data about utilization, and while using medical records data for purposes of quality assurance and cost containment. There seems to be no record of problems arising out of any misuse of confidential medical information by either the nonprofit or the commercial health insurance industry.

Self-Insurance Narrows the Options

An employer or union might someday regret its decision to self-insure and self-administer health coverage because a consequence of the decision is to narrow the options for future directions in benefit programs, in at least two ways.

First, one must not underestimate the size of the commitment which a group must make in staffing, data processing, and overhead when taking on the assignments that are ordinarily performed by a health insurer. A competent capacity to process, to review and pay claims, to keep track of eligibility, to adjudicate disputes, and to develop new or altered benefit patterns requires a considerable long-term investment in professional and technical personnel, computerization, and support services.

The costs of that investment are likely to be much higher than initially projected, if only because the environment for health coverage is getting ever more complex in terms of regulatory requirements, consumer expectations, and the very nature of modern medical care. It is therefore quite conceivable that within just a few years, the group that chose to self-insure and self-administer will begin to question whether it is indeed realizing the savings it had anticipated. At the same time, questions may be accumulating as to whether the program is achieving its objectives in terms of cost containment, employee satisfaction, and so on.

However, because of the substantial commitment of resources, to say nothing of prestige and pride, which the group makes in developing its self-insurance capacity, any major change becomes most onerous. It is surely easier to change insurance carriers on the basis of dissatisfaction with costs or performance than to disband or significantly cut back an entire department of a large company or a union welfare fund. Indeed, the group may be virtually locked into persisting with the *status quo*.

Second, health coverage is in a considerable state of flux. A case in point is the burgeoning of HMOs, which a combination of federal and state laws, consumer demands, and common sense obliges most benefit plans to make available to members. One could presume that because HMOs tend to combine significant cost savings with good quality services, this development would not be opposed by most self-insured groups. Experience suggests, however, that many such groups resist giving their members an HMO option, probably because the group thereby effectively loses control over those persons' health coverage and benefits administration.

The at least partial incompatibility of HMOs with self-insurance and self-administration is only part of the story. Insurers frequently bring into the market—or offer experimentally on an extracontractual basis—new and different kinds of benefits. For example, several Blue Cross plans and commercial insurers are currently trying out approaches to covering such services as non-traditional maternity programs, hospices, alcoholism rehabilitation programs, voluntary second surgical opinion programs, home health care programs, and the like. They are doing important developmental work and thereby accepting a measure of risk.

For the most part, this kind of innovation appears to be beyond the reach of self-insured, self-administered programs. Not only do they usually lack the scope to carry out the necessary developmental and implementing work, but they would tend to be chary of offering a benefit to employees if they might later have to withdraw it, or if they couldn't deliver it uniformly.

Conclusion

It is not surprising that some major purchasers of health insurance coverage are frustrated and impatient with constantly rising benefit expenditures, complaints from members about service and coverage, and what appears to be high overhead. In some environments, the available health insurance carriers may appear to be slow in responding to a host of new demands and challenges. Consultants may be urging seemingly plausible new approaches, including self-insured and self-administered health benefit programs.

The purpose of this presentation has been to suggest that while these propositions may appear attractive—and may even offer some short-term advantages—employers, unions, and other large purchasers would be well advised to consider carefully whether they are prepared for the possible consequences of administering and insuring benefit programs themselves. Health insurance is a highly competitive market, with nonprofit prepayment plans and commercial insurers vying with one another to obtain their shares. Groups have powerful alternatives to self-insurance, if they exercise their purchasing power effectively.

U. S. Administrators

Samuel X. Kaplan

At last some corporations and unions show signs of focusing their interest on the inflationary crises in the nation's health care system. I say "some" because many corporate benefits personnel still believe insurance company rhetoric that evaluating usual and customary charges is what a cost containment and utilization review system is all about. I say "some" also because many corporate labor relations personnel and union leaders prefer a pay-as-billed system, the kind that avoids any "heat" from the employee/member who is used to having somebody else pay all of a bill as charged, less any deductibles, coinsurance, or maximums. But attention is finally turning toward questions of fundamental change, toward putting a stop to the alarming increases in health care costs which are estimated for next year at more than double the amount spent only five years ago.

Why No Action?

Incredibly, no one has really cared about the soaring costs of medical care—I mean cared enough to insist on *effective action*. Neither the nation's foremost statemen, nor the government, nor the insurance companies, nor most corporations and unions, and certainly not the providers. Why? Because sombody else is paying the bill.

Somebody else always pays, so almost everyone accepts the current condition of the health care delivery system in the United States as an inevitable and insurmountable fact of life. Like death itself, it is regarded with grave and stoic indifference. Overutilization of services, unnecessary medical and surgical procedures, unreasonable charges, and deterioration of the quality of care are generally ignored or overlooked because somebody else pays and nearly everyone is benefiting.

The insurance companies are benefiting. Increased costs of health care lead to escalating reserves available for investment. With insurance company charges based on a percentage of premium or claims, the higher the health care expenditures the greater their income.

Some consumers are benefiting. They go along with a provider who charges for unnecessary or never performed procedures but waives all portions of the bill normally payable by the consumer.

Some corporate and union personnel with benefit responsibilities are also benefiting. They shy away from any study of what can be accomplished in cost containment and utilization review. They need only float along in the mainstream of insurance company rhetoric and advertising, and they can point to many other corporations and unions and truthfully say, "We're in no worse position than they are."

Many broker/consultants benefit. Those reimbursed on a percentage-of-premium basis ride the tails of inflationary health care costs. And many of those on a fee basis find it easier to ride along with the insurance industry, thereby eliminating the need to think, investigate, probe, conceive, and report.

Finally, the providers—does anyone doubt that the providers are benefiting under the current condition? Note, I said "condition," not "system"—I do not believe there is anything wrong with the system if properly controlled; however, there is a great deal wrong with the current condition of the system.

Some say that almost everyone accepts the current condition because everyone benefits under it. Do the insurance companies and service corporations really care? Do they have the guts to do something about it? Maybe they care, but they have not and apparently will not take on the incompetent, the poorly trained, the overutilizing, or the underutilizing provider; nor will they assume responsibility for establishing and enforcing standards and criteria for health care.

What Can Be Done?

First, there must be a realization by corporations and unions of what is the cost of health care. According to a Louis Harris poll conducted for Chicago's

Mount Sinai Hospital, almost 50 percent of the senior officers in charge of corporate employee benefits for 51 Fortune Double 500 companies in the Chicago area were "unsure" of the cost per employee of their companies' health insurance plans—either in dollar terms or in percentages of salary. Even fewer knew their companies' health care costs for the previous five years. Twelve percent of those surveyed thought their annual health care costs were less than $100 per employee per year. "It's difficult to escape the conclusion," the November 1977 survey observes, "that [the companies] might do a more effective job of controlling health care costs if they knew what costs are now and how they have changed over the last few years." Another striking finding was the broad consensus among the sample that no organization, company or institution involved with health care was doing even a reasonably good job of controlling health care costs. The criticisms were directed particularly at hospitals, physicians and the American Medical Association . . . "whose job it should be (in the eyes of corporate benefits officers) to do much more than they are doing now." To even think that most hospitals, physicians or the AMA would take effective voluntary action toward a cost containment effort is as ludicrous as setting the fox to guard the henhouse. However, it was not only the hospitals, physicians and the AMA that were found lacking for their efforts. Consumers, employers, the federal government and labor unions also came in for their fair share of criticism for doing little or nothing to control health care costs.

The corporation or union who does care about costs and quality can do something about both. Traditional insurance industry approaches to health care are no longer relevant. Corporations, unions, and multiple-employer trusts who want to cut costs need self-insurance and they need effective claims administration through a cost containment and utilization review system. Let us examine these concepts in detail.

Advantages of Self-Insurance

There are three basic reasons for the relatively recent surge of interest in self-insurance.

1. The financial squeeze in which many companies find themselves has been a major contributor to the interest in self-insured plans. Financial officers of corporations, cognizant of the large amounts being spent on premium taxes, and also aware of the reserves being held by insurance companies and service plans, frequently stimulate benefits managers to investigate alternatives to the fully-insured health plan.

This awareness of the reserve and premium tax considerations on the part of the financial officers frequently comes from consultants, brokers and health plan administrators who use the promise of savings from self-insurance as a sales tool or "door-opener."

2. In the past, there has been reluctance on the part of many corporations to adopt a self-insured health plan because of the fear of legal problems with state regulatory agencies. However, ERISA has a provision

which prohibits a state from considering a self-insured plan to be an insurance company for the purpose of regulation. This removes the major legal reason for not self-insuring.

3.   Many corporations have been reluctant to assume the administrative and claims services which carriers provide. Even those corporations which were on a draft book basis relied on the carrier for assistance on problem claims. Now, however, insurers sell administrative services separately, without the risk portion of "insurance package." Such services are also available from companies which specialize in administering self-insured plans. Although there are several terms used in describing a situation where the insurer sells administrative and claims services independently of the risk portion of the package, the most commonly used phrase is "administrative services only" or "ASO." A term beginning to be heard more frequently is "administrative services contract" or "ASC" which encompasses more services by the administrator.

The advantages of self-insurance are, simply stated, tax exemption of investment earnings, elimination of state premium taxes, elimination of many carrier charges, wider investment possibilities, and greater flexibility in contributions.

For a single employer, self-insuring health and life insurance benefits through a trust is not a tax loophole or legal gimmick. On the contrary, Section 501(c)(9) of the Internal Revenue Code says that employer contributions to the trust are deductible as a cost of doing business. Also, the earnings on the reserves of the fund are tax-exempt. And the employee may not be taxed on contributions made by the employer to the fund. Additionally, there are no minimum contribution requirements and no limits on allowable contributions.

Self-insuring health and insurance benefits also offers four potential areas of savings related to insurance company retention formulas. First is the savings on state premium taxes. Premiums paid to an insurance company are taxed by all states. Naturally, this tax is passed on to the policyholder as an item in the retention. State premium taxes range from 2 to 4 percent of premium, mostly on net premium but occasionally on the gross. Unfortunately, unlike other items which tend to decrease as the premium increases, state premium taxes remain constant and may constitute the largest single item in the retention. Contributions to a 501(c)(9) trust, since the enactment of ERISA, are not subject to state premium taxes. Some states have attempted to include these trusts under tax laws. Under Connecticut law, for example, employee welfare benefit plans had to pay a tax. The amount of tax was 2.75 percent of all benefits paid through a self-insurance mechanism to participant and beneficiaries residing in the state. However, a declaratory judgment handed down by a U.S. District Court two months ago declares this law void and unenforceable as it applies to ERISA-covered plans. The decision also enjoins the State Tax Commissioner from assessing or collecting such taxes. The states' power to tax an ERISA-covered plan is preempted by ERISA Sec. 415 which supercedes any and all state laws insofar as they may relate to any employee benefit plan. The decision says that the phrase "any and all" in the Act plainly indicates an intention to reach every state statute that fits the description of relating to employee benefit plans. The

Connecticut law is seen as such a statute, particularly since it is not merely a general taxing provision that "catches employee benefit plans within its wide sweep" but also a statute "specifically directed at such plans exclusively." The decision also rejects Connecticut's contention that preemption is not necessary to accomplish ERISA's objective of insulating plans from potentially conflicting state regulatory requirements. The court says that "the power to tax entails the power to regulate as well."

For now, at least, it appears that states will not be able to levy a tax on a self-insured mechanism used for employee welfare benefit plans.

The second potential area of cost savings in the retention formula is an item that is called "profit" by the stock companies. Whatever the service corporations and mutuals prefer to call it, this "item" is built into the retention formula—neither service corporations, mutuals, nor stock companies are charitable institutions. Self-insurance eliminates this retention charge. Third, self-insurance eliminates charges allocated by insurance companies and service corporations to advertising, promotion, and sales expenses.

Fourth, self-insurance eliminates or drastically reduces monies assigned to contingency or similar reserves. This means that the employer has use of money which approximates 25 percent of annual premium—a major reason to consider self-insurance.

Even though there are various arrangements available to minimize the impact of reserves on a fully or partially insured health plan, they are not as direct or "clean" as the elimination of reserves under the self-insured program.

In deciding whether the corporation should establish reserves for a self-insured health care program, it may be helpful to consider why insurers establish reserves. Among the reasons are:

1. So they can have assets on which interest is being earned.

2. Because state insurance departments require reserves be held.

3. In order to have money to pay claims which were incurred before the employer terminated the contract.

Note that the only reason why an employer might wish to hold reserves—to minimize the effect of fluctuations in claims payments—is not listed. That is because insurers usually pool or reinsure against exessive claims liabilities. Employers can also buy stop-loss coverage to protect themselves against excessive claims.

Most self-insured health plans do not have reserves. However, if the corporation decides to establish reserves for its self-insured health care plan, it should consider establishing a trust to hold those reserves. Indeed, Sec. 403(a) of ERISA requires that all assets of an employee benefit plan be held by a trust. Therefore, if a self-insured plan is going to establish reserves, it would appear that a simple book reserve will not be suitable; a 501(c)(9) trust would appear to be the most satisfactory vehicle.

Life insurance company and casualty company reserves are used to meet extraordinary calls on life risks and the specific casualty risk. But the amount and assignment of reserves accumulated by a self-insured trust can be applied to whichever risk requires the money, and management is free to decide whether or not to accumulate large reserves.

Two potential cost savings not found in the retention formula concern claims reserves: first, in the area of investments; second, the flexibility of cash flows. Insured and self-insured plans both invest reserves held to meet ongoing and future claims. Insurance company assets are usually invested in a limited range of securities, but the self-insured trust is free to make broad-range investments, limited only by the fiduciary responsibilities of the trustees. Investment returns can thus be substantially different. An increase in earnings of 1 percent per year over a ten to twenty year period, for example, will save 5 to 18 percent in claims reserves, depending on how the reserves are built up. And, happily, unlike insurance company invested reserves, earnings of 501(c)(9) trust reserves are tax-free.

Cash flow flexibility is another important advantage of self-insurance. Under insured plans, premiums usually are paid at specified intervals, but self-insurance allows flexibility in the timing of contributions. The same holds true for contributions to reserves. Under insured plans, carriers prescribe reserve formulas for each specific risk, but self-insured corporations maintain complete control over reserve levels.

Disadvantages of Self-Insurance

Cost savings aside for the moment, self-insurance is not without potential disadvantages. Let us consider the problems: the element of risk, administrative headaches related to terminated employees, the possibility of joint administration with unions, and the threat to employee relations.

For most risks covered by employee health benefits, the size of the group need not be large to make self-insurance feasible. The rule of thumb has been that groups over 1,000 employees are sufficient. Today, there are a number of companies offering specific and aggregate stop-loss protection for groups wishing to self-insure with as few as 50 employees. Averages of workdays lost to illness, accident, and hospitalization work out about the same for several hundred employees as for several thousand. Smaller groups will, of course, experience greater fluctuations from the average, but not enough to impair self-insurance.

The ideal benefit for self-insurance is characterized by high frequency of claims and low cost per individual claim. The smaller the amount of each claim, the smaller the impact of claims above the projected number. However, as the group increases in size, each claim payment is smaller relative to the total amount of claim payments. As a result, the element of risk in self-insurance trusts is minimal.

As for administrative headaches related to terminated employees, it is true that a 501(c)(9) trust cannot continue to cover persons who cease to be employees of the sponsoring corporation. But this potential disadvantage can be mitigated by an arrangement with a carrier to provide conversion privileges.

Regarding the danger of catastrophe resulting in enormous, unplanned-for claims, the problem can be either set aside, resolved by reinsurance, or allayed by accumulation of reserves.

Another potential disadvantage to an employer is that unions could demand joint benefit administration. Benefits provided through a 501(c) (9) trust in part for union-represented employees might result in union demands for a board of trustees comprised equally of union and employer representatives.

On the question of threats to employee relations, employee ill will could result from claims that are questioned or refused. Normally directed toward the insurance company, this ill will could be turned on the employer. This is a frequently cited advantage of the insured plan in that the insurer acts as a buffer to "protect" the employer from unions, doctors and disgruntled employees. The degree to which this "buffer" is effective varies from company to company, and depends on the relative sophistication of the union representatives and/or employees.

As a practical matter, however, the third party buffer argument is invalid. Sec. 503 of ERISA specifically states that "every employee benefit plan" shall provide participants with a reasonable opportunity for "a full and fair review" of denied claims by the named fiduciary. This means that the corporate benefit plan administrator (who will probably be the named fiduciary) will be the scapegoat for a denied claim whether a plan is insured or self-insured.

None of the above potential difficulties is sufficient, in my opinion, to outweigh the preponderant cost advantages of self-insurance. Indeed, very much the same list of advantages and disadvantages held—and still holds—for self-insured pension plans, but most pension plans today are self-insured.

A final question concerns the administration of self-insured plans. This should not be a problem. First, let us enumerate the services which the carrier usually provides under a fully-insured program.

1. *Enrollment* presents little problem to the self-insured plan since the employer usually handles most of the details irrespective of the method of funding.

2. *Contracts.* Under a self-insured plan, there are no insurance contracts to be filed with the state insurance departments. This can prove to be a decided advantage; more than one state has required meaningless phrases or provisions which do little but frustrate those who are attempting to develop a relatively uniform national contract.

There will, of course, need to be contracts between the employer and those who are administering the self-insured program, but these contracts are not subject to the same type of state regulation as the insurance contract, and therefore there is no outside interference.

3. *Booklets and Certificates.* Since there is no insurance in a self-insured plan, certificates are not required. Nevertheless, it is important that the employees have information about the benefit program under which they are covered. The absence of an insurance policy makes this especially important.

The self-insured plan is not exempt from the ERISA requirements that the employee benefit plan must be communicated to the employee in a clear, easy-to-understand manner.

4. *Actuarial and Legal Services.* Actuarial services include supervision of underwriting and rate making. Neither of these can be eliminated in a self-insured plan. Knowing the cost of the health coverage is necessary for budgeting and for negotiations. It is also important to accurately determine the cost of the self-insured plan in order to arrive at the proper contribution which the employer will make on behalf of employees who select coverage under a qualified health maintenance organization, in accordance with Sec. 1310 of the HMO Act.

Should the consultant provide the actuarial services, or is it better to include "actuarial" as part of the ASO contract? In making such a decision, the benefits manager will want to consider the background and experience of those who will be doing the work. An actuary who tends to specialize in pension work may not be able to bring the same level of competence to health care actuarial work as an actuary who spends all of his time in the health benefits field.

Turning to legal services, it should be noted that most insurers take the position that they cannot sell legal services. Under an insured or partially-insured plan, the carrier's legal staff defends claims and tries to cut through the legal haze surrounding contracts because it is part of the total package which an insurer provides to policyholders.

However, if the insurer is merely the agent for paying claims and is providing a few other services, it is generally agreed that those "other services" cannot include legal help.

5. *Conversion* of self-insured contracts can be a knotty problem unless the employer purchases conversion coverage from a carrier which offers the product in connection with a stop-loss contract. Recently, some carriers have started offering conversion coverage without a stop-loss contract.

6. *Claims Handling, Review and Cost Containment* have, in the past, been the main obstacles for an employer to hurdle before becoming self-insured. It is important that the administrator selected has a proven system to review the appropriateness and necessity of treatment and will act as an ombudsman for the patient.

We have seen that the services usually provided by the carrier can as easily be provided, with certain advantages, under an ASO or ASC contract. In either case, the cost is about equal to the retention item for these services in an insured plan.

Cost Containment and Utilization Review

Savings on self-insured plans under a 501(c) (9) trust will amount to 10 to 15 percent annually. But savings will be even greater—another 15 to 20 percent greater—when the self-insurance program is coupled with an effective claims administrator who has implemented an operative, honest-to-goodness cost containment and utilization review system. Such an administrator rises above the simple routines of claims processing and check writing and gets down to nitty-gritty responsibilities for assuring (1) that charges are made only for services actually provided; (2) that services provided are actually necessary; and (3) that the services provided are of high quality. In other words, the administrator assumes the triple obligation of offering protection for the patient, service to the provider, and fiscal responsibility to the third party payor.

Effective claims administration is divided into two distinct functions: the mechanical task of claims processing, payment, accounting, data collection and tabulation, and the critical task of claims review, which includes provider activity analysis, quality control, medical audit, and peer review. These two interrelated and interdependent functions must be contained in a total system. That system should be responsive to the provider who performs according to established standards and guidelines, should impose a minimum of constraints on his activity, and should also be capable of identifying and dealing quickly and effectively with the provider who does not perform according to those standards and guidelines—especially with the provider who attempts to subvert the system or manipulate the health care consumer for personal gain. In short, the system should be responsive to the cooperative and capable provider, but be able to significantly reduce abuse, overutilization, and underutilization.

An effective claims review system, we have found, begins with the establishment of a model treatment program (MTP) which establishes criteria for over 4,000 medical diagnoses. Utilizing a sophisticated computer system, the MTP reviews every single claim, checking each for such items as the reasonableness of the treatment in relation to the diagnosis, age and sex compatibility of patient to diagnosis and treatment, the place of service, surgery follow-up days, number of days in hospital, and so forth. MTP's computer system flags all claims that appear to surpass established criteria.

Human judgment resolves the questions raised by the computer. But the computer, make no mistake about it, is the workhorse of the MTP system. It stores huge amounts of data that relate diagnoses to suitable treatments and indicates the frequency of acceptable treatments. It analyzes a patient's history and pinpoints overtreatment, undertreatment, and mistreatment. It analyzes costs, compares medical procedures of one provider with another, reviews hospitalization records, checks ancillary services. Meanwhile, it continues to process claims.

In the case of hospitalized patients, MTP exercises both prospective and retrospective review. Should the patient have been hospitalized for the given diagnosis? Were there any duplicated services? And most important, did the length of stay exceed the average for this diagnosis? Invariably, the lower the bed occupancy rate in hospitals, the longer the stay for *all* diagnoses. For ambulatory patients, the most common and costly abuses are overuse of injections, excessive office visits, and excessive diagnostic procedures. The most common and costly surgical abuse is—you guessed it—far too many surgeries. MTP catches the violations and the violators.

In short, an effective claims review system must be comprehensive. You need a model treatment program based on the best and most complete set of health standards and criteria. You need a sophisticated computer system to implement MTP. And you need administrators motivated to eliminate plan abuses and to cut costs—without sacrificing the quality of delivered care or denying consumers access to the system. To reduce a provider's charges and have the patient pay the amount of the reduction is *not* a cost containment program. In a cost containment program, the administrator must hold harmless the patient against any attempt to collect fees for those services determined to be inappropriate or unnecessary.

From our experience and the experience of our clients, an effective cost containment and utilization review system is the only feasible way to administer large health care plans. Without an MTP system, you remain at the mercy of provider abuse and incompetence. With such a system, you maintain high standards of quality, and you virtually eliminate plan abuses. Also, with such a system, you can make the move to self-funding with confidence.

What Is the Answer?

Today, self-insurance is working for many large companies, even without an effective cost containment and utilization review system. These companies are realizing the 10 to 15 percent savings that result from self-insuring. But companies such as H. F. Ahmanson, Del Monte, Hunt-Wesson, Johns-Manville, and others are enjoying savings of 25 to 30 percent because of effective cost containment and utilization review systems.

In private, the carriers admit they have no real power over the system— that they exercise no control over providers or provider practices. They claim that this is really the fault of their policyholders because they are only following their policyholders' orders. But, they have to *appear* to be doing something. So different insurance companies are taking different routes in attempting to solve our monumental health care problems. Some companies are promoting health education and physical fitness and some are lobbying for government controls such as the extension of PSROs for private patients and state commissions for prospective hospital budget review. (I wonder if they would be so eager for federal controls if part of the package was to be federal regulation of the insurance industry!) Some are advocating more deductibles and coinsurance and some are only advertising their merits.

But these so-called solutions will not solve America's monumental health care problems. If the insurance companies became operative PSROs—as every administrator should be—that would go a long way toward controlling provider and patient abuses. But the carriers don't have the stomach for it. Meanwhile, the cost of corporation health care continues to skyrocket.

Self-insuring is the answer. With or without insurance company administration, self-insurance will reduce costs 10 to 15 percent. In my opinion, not more than 20 percent of companies or unions want an able administrator, but if you really want to reduce health care costs, self-insurance and an effective administrator will provide the best available combination for effective action.

United Mine Workers of America Health and Retirement Funds

Stephen C. Caulfield

The United Mine Workers of America Health and Retirement Funds have been a self-insured provider of physician and hospital benefits to bituminous coal workers, dependents, pensioners, and survivors since 1947. During all this time, the funds have defined their role as a discriminating purchaser of care, not simply a payer of medical bills. Accordingly, we instituted in 1947 a system of claims review which has become increasingly refined over the years. By 1977, at which time the funds covered over 800,000 beneficiaries in all fifty states, an automated data system had been implemented which served to regularize and further refine the claims review system. Unfortunately, this system is unlikely to survive the 1978 national bituminous coal wage agreement that sharply curtailed the funds' health benefit responsibilities. Nevertheless, our experience of more than thirty years can provide some detailed procedural suggestions as well as some evaluative insights to companies and unions now considering in-house claims review under a self-insured health benefits plan.

Table 1
Health Service Card Population by Age Group and Sex by Region and Field Service Office, July 1, 1977

Region; Field Service Office	Total	Male				Female			
		0–14	15–44	45–64	65 +	0–14	15–44	45–64	65 +
Beckley	161,841	23,822	36,591	13,712	7,659	22,559	34,380	15,417	7,701
Beckley	61,610	8,633	13,323	5,360	3,418	8,262	12,503	6,431	3,680
Logan	63,811	9,935	14,994	5,204	2,417	9,319	14,045	5,650	2,247
Cabin Creek	36,420	5,254	8,274	3,148	1,824	4,978	7,832	3,336	1,774
Central Appalachian	184,189	25,236	39,334	16,029	11,321	23,837	37,465	19,687	11,280
Big Stone Gap	29,115	4,022	6,415	2,531	1,507	3,899	6,159	3,007	1,575
Welch	43,878	6,334	9,806	3,752	2,139	6,040	9,082	4,453	2,272
Middlesboro	20,495	1,954	3,063	1,988	2,814	1,803	2,902	3,147	2,824
Allen	35,246	5,181	7,518	3,182	1,874	4,806	7,274	3,625	1,786
Richlands	38,716	5,651	9,334	3,038	1,571	5,277	8,864	3,464	1,517
Jenkins	16,739	2,094	3,198	1,538	1,416	2,012	3,184	1,991	1,306
Birmingham	48,266	6,087	9,665	4,107	3,924	5,710	9,469	5,352	3,952
Birmingham	48,266	6,087	9,665	4,107	3,924	5,710	9,469	5,352	3,952

Western	32,670	4,473	6,430	2,461	3,164	4,232	5,707	3,157	3,046
Denver	15,701	1,702	2,598	1,265	2,199	1,666	2,385	1,757	2,129
Price	16,969	2,771	3,832	1,196	965	2,566	3,322	1,400	917
Johnstown	104,332	11,242	18,843	10,799	11,206	10,767	16,314	13,929	11,232
Johnstown	63,102	7,448	12,013	6,122	6,006	7,266	10,437	7,856	5,954
Washington	24,161	2,141	3,898	2,885	3,066	1,965	3,356	3,750	3,100
New Kensington	17,069	1,653	2,932	1,792	2,134	1,536	2,521	2,323	2,178
Midwest	122,956	16,363	26,244	10,032	8,668	15,138	24,713	11,408	10,390
Evansville	55,306	7,605	12,117	4,551	3,468	7,004	11,552	5,114	3,895
Benton	41,556	5,717	9,162	3,170	2,604	5,360	8,504	3,482	3,557
Springfield	17,999	2,188	3,682	1,585	1,548	2,043	3,350	1,850	1,753
Fort Smith	8,095	853	1,283	726	1,048	731	1,307	962	1,185
Morgantown	158,154	20,288	33,075	14,437	11,955	19,345	29,623	17,610	11,821
Morgantown	55,037	7,363	11,422	5,356	3,375	7,156	10,885	6,125	3,355
Wheeling	67,725	9,353	15,520	4,955	4,793	8,893	13,334	6,354	4,523
Uniontown	35,392	3,572	6,133	4,126	3,787	3,296	5,404	5,131	3,943
Other	427	20	22	33	55	12	30	62	193
ALL REGIONS	812,835	107,531	170,204	71,610	57,952	101,600	157,701	86,622	59,615

Manual Claims Review

Because of the wide dispersal of UMWA Funds' beneficiaries, our first review and control efforts were implemented more or less independently by each of a series of regional offices (numbering twenty-nine when the system was at its largest). The efforts at cost and quality control took a number of forms. Each office developed a list of participating providers (physicians, hospitals, and clinics) based on staff perceptions of beneficiaries' need for services and of the costs and quality of those providers' services. The offices also undertook active support of resource development where necessary through offering staff assistance and financing to group practices, clinics, and hospitals. Control mechanisms included an administrative requirement for prior approval of certain health care procedures, staff review of cost-based reimbursements, as well as a drug benefit for chronic conditions limited to a specific formulary and administered through a very limited list of mail-out vendors.

The review of claims received was conducted manually for many years. This review used only the information and standards developed by the regional office involved. Reviewers made value judgments about costs and quality as reflected in individual claims. Payment mechanisms emphasized prepayment through an average cost-based, fee-for-time retainer for ambulatory care and through cost-based per diems for inpatient care.

While this conceptual approach to benefits management was and is sound, it suffered in practice from the lack of uniform and detailed data collection and retrieval and of uniform policies and procedures. It therefore led to ad hoc value judgments that changed over time and across regions, causing considerable variation in programs and questionable levels of control. To correct these problems, the Health and Retirement Funds sought to automate their claims-processing system. The automated claims system including a Surveillance and Utilization Review Subsystem (or SUR), is designed to provide accurate data on the nature of claims paid and, more significantly, to provide management information regarding the provision of health care.

Automated Claims Review

The process of automating the claims system forced a degree of rigor on the cost containment efforts that had previously been exercised in an ad hoc fashion. SUR provides us with detailed beneficiary and provider data, with the data necessary for procedure and fee control, and with some of the prerequisites for utilization review and quality control.

Beneficiary information was automated to create an on-line record of each of the 280,000 cardholders and each of their dependents (total population 813,000) by benefit coverage, eligibility period, age, sex, address, and cash benefit payment records. Health payment records by beneficiary are compiled separately and maintained off line. This beneficiary data base enables us to identify age- and sex-specific concentrations geographically down to zip code levels (see table 1).

Providers of health and hospital care, whose numbers had been limited through a closed list of participating physicians and hospitals, were placed into a computer provider file. When all providers actually paid were identified, it became apparent that the perception of a highly limited provider list was in error. Still, although the provider file was significantly larger than anticipated, the funds were dealing with fewer than 20,000 billing physicians, clinics, hospitals, and pharmacies to serve all beneficiaries in all the states. Further, because beneficiaries were concentrated in seven states, it became clear that the majority of services were rendered through a group of only about twenty clinics and group practices. Thus, the funds had considerable influence—40 percent or more of patient load—on these providers that delivered the majority of services. Nonparticipating physicians that often provided care to beneficiaries were on the provider file in a "stop-pay" status. The provider file enables us to identify providers by type by region (see table 2). Payment data provides volume of business information, useful for many purposes including investigations of possible abuse.

Procedure controls, which had focused under the manual system on prior approvals, were automated in two ways. First, each provider had specific authorizations built into his or her file. Operating as we do in rural areas, we have had some experience of physicians functioning beyond their expertise. As a general rule we authorize no surgery or orthopedics for general practitioners. Second, the procedure file identified all procedures by Current Procedural Terminology (CPT 3) codes as either covered benefit, covered benefit requiring prior authorization, or not a covered benefit.

For purposes of fee control, we first developed a system of procedure-specific fee edits for twelve classes of physician provider (e.g., general practitioner, board-certified radiologist, etc.) based on limited empirical data, regional "guestimates," and relative value scales. This proved to be cumbersome and unworkable; we are moving to a procedure-specific fee edit for excessive charges. We have avoided the Medicare profile approach.

Utilization review under the manual system had been limited to aggregate statistical data by region for length of stay by diagnosis, rates of admission, days per 1,000, and costs. Patterns of practice for specific providers and patterns of utilization for individuals were not available. This information is obviously essential if one intends to manage a limited-market, closed system, and thus was a basic requirement for our automated system. We now have the capacity to profile by month or quarter inpatient and outpatient provider practice with regard to our beneficiaries and beneficiary utilization. (Table 3 shows sample printout information.)

Quality control in health care, particularly from a claims payment perspective, is at best tentative and usually illusory. With a highly decentralized regional office system, the funds had access to local hearsay knowledge to influence the selection of participating providers—such items as "no one will scrub with him," "he uses injectable steroids for virtually everything," and so on. This information, when corroborated by colleagues, can be useful in limiting the participating program, but we wondered if we could develop, through a claims-based data system, some retrospective measures of quality, particularly of ambulatory care. Tables 4 and 5 describe the variables currently used and

Table 2
Provider Resources by Type of Region and Field Service Office

Region and field service office[a]	Office total	Practitioner (1)	Group practice (2)	Home health (3)	Independent laboratory (4)	Family planning clinic (5)	Medical clinic (6)
Central Appalachian Regional Office							
11	536	412	2	2	4	X	24
12	484	313	40	7	5	X	39
14	1,623	1,192	159	12	13	X	30
16	890	696	50	5	8	X	14
18	691	502	71	1	4	1	18
19	103	61	3	4	X	X	8
Total	4,327	3,176	325	31	34	1	133
Birmingham							
22	4,234	3,088	467	6	31	X	9
Western							
32	3,990	2,990	324	X	50	1	2
34	934	703	87	X	12	X	X
Total	4,924	3,693	411	X	62	1	2
Johnstown							
42	3,757	2,655	274	11	55	19	18
44	1,658	1,257	166	6	16	4	4
46	481	340	40	8	1	X	6
Total	5,896	4,252	480	25	72	23	28
Midwest							
52	2,497	1,854	207	6	23	X	36
54	1,177	822	137	3	18	X	2
56	1,316	993	102	2	7	X	X
58	1,314	946	130	X	12	X	X
Total	6,304	4,615	576	11	60	X	38
Morgantown							
62	1,005	503	34	8	7	6	282
64	5,075	3,776	288	8	53	38	54
66	315	187	24	2	2	X	1
Total	6,395	4,466	346	18	62	44	337
Beckley							
72	285	191	16	X	3	1	7
74	319	242	22	2	X	X	9
76	509	369	42	2	7	X	9
Total	1,113	802	80	4	10	1	25
Funds Total	33,193	24,092	2,685	95	331	70	572

SOURCE: Hard Copy Regional Alphabetic Microfiche, 4/03/77
[a]Field service offices identified by numerical code.

Rehabilitation center (7)	Medical supply (8)	Out-patient hospital (9)	In-patient hospital (10)	Skilled nursing facility (11)	Custodial care facility (12)	Pharmacy (13)	Ambulance (14)
X	13	31	36	3	X	1	8
2	21	11	26	5	X	3	12
3	31	50	73	13	12	7	28
X	17	32	33	6	X	7	21
X	1	34	41	X	2	3	13
X	2	6	X	3	X	6	10
5	85	164	209	30	14	27	92
6	88	237	244	9	X	5	44
X	63	258	260	X	X	1	41
X	27	49	45	X	X	X	11
X	90	307	305	X	X	1	52
3	74	258	280	24	X	22	64
18	46	48	50	6	1	7	29
X	30	13	14	8	X	X	21
21	150	319	344	38	1	29	114
13	48	136	139	10	X	2	23
X	42	57	59	3	X	1	33
1	60	65	65	3	X	X	18
X	35	88	88	X	X	X	15
14	185	346	351	16	X	3	89
1	26	35	42	10	1	6	44
13	92	309	303	14	1	19	107
1	14	9	16	16	X	6	37
15	132	353	361	40	2	31	188
X	17	11	9	2	X	9	19
X	10	12	10	X	1	2	9
1	30	11	11	3	X	5	19
1	57	34	30	5	1	16	47
62	787	1,760	1,844	138	18	112	626

Table 3
Individual Provider Profile: Items Paid During Quarter Ending 03/31/77

```
REF NO                    HSID=            NAME=I                   ATTENDING DR=          BIRTHDATE              SEX=F  MEDICARE 1 ACCIDENT NO
PROV NAME=DRS                                       PROV NO=                                                           ATT DR PROV NO=
DIAGNOSIS=GENERAL MED EXAM NEC                                                      VST IN= 0 VST OTH= 1         CHECK DATE 02/04/77
LINE 31   PROCEDURE=OFFICE VISIT=LIMITED SERVICE, TYPE OF PT. UNSPECIFIED   QUANTITY          1
          SERVICE DATE  11/16/76          PLACE OF SERVICE=0                                                    CHARGE        $10.00

TOTAL CHARGES    $10.00                   MEDICARE PYMT         $0.00   INS PYMT                  $0.00   TOTAL PAID    $10.00


REF NO                    HSID=            NAME=                    ATTENDING DR=        B BIRTHDATE              SEX=F  MEDICARE 1 ACCIDENT NO
PROV NAME=DRS                                       PROV NO=                                                           ATT DR PROV NO=
DIAGNOSIS=SEBORRHEIC DERMATITIS                                                     VST IN= 0 VST OTH= 1         CHECK DATE 02/04/77
LINE 41   PROCEDURE=OFFICE VISIT=LIMITED SERVICE, TYPE OF PT. UNSPECIFIED   QUANTITY          1
          SERVICE DATE  11/30/76          PLACE OF SERVICE=0                                                    CHARGE        $10.00

TOTAL CHARGES    $10.00                   MEDICARE PYMT         $0.00   INS PYMT                  $0.00   TOTAL PAID    $10.00


REF NO                    HSID=            NAME=                    ATTENDING DR=I       B BIRTHDATE              SEX=F  MEDICARE 1 ACCIDENT NO
PROV NAME=                                          PROV NO=                                                           ATT DR PROV NO=
DIAGNOSIS=SEBORRHEIC DERMATITIS                                                     VST IN= 0 VST OTH= 1         CHECK DATE 02/04/77
LINE 41   PROCEDURE=OFFICE VISIT=LIMITED SERVICE, TYPE OF PT. UNSPECIFIED   QUANTITY          1
          SERVICE DATE  11/30/76          PLACE OF SERVICE=0                                                    CHARGE        $10.00

TOTAL CHARGES    $10.00                   MEDICARE PYMT         $0.00   INS PYMT                  $0.00   TOTAL PAID    $10.00


REF NO                    HSID=            NAME=                    ATTENDING DR=        A BIRTHDATE              SEX=F  MEDICARE 1 ACCIDENT NO
PROV NAME=DRS                                       PROV NO=                                                           ATT DR PROV NO=
DIAGNOSIS=ACUTE BRONCHIOLITIS (4891)                                               VST IN= 0 VST OTH= 1         CHECK DATE 02/04/77
LINE 21   PROCEDURE=OFFICE VISIT=LIMITED SERVICE, TYPE OF PT. UNSPECIFIED   QUANTITY          1
          SERVICE DATE  11/30/76          PLACE OF SERVICE=0                                                    CHARGE        $10.00

LINE 22   PROCEDURE=THERAPEUTIC INJECTION, ANTIBIOTIC                       QUANTITY          1
          SERVICE DATE  11/30/76          PLACE OF SERVICE=0                                                    CHARGE         $8.00

TOTAL CHARGES    $18.00                   MEDICARE PYMT         $0.00   INS PYMT                  $0.00   TOTAL PAID    $18.00
```

Table 4
SUR Quality Review Variables, Provider

Health Care Setting	Variables	Objectives	
		Quality	Cost
Ambulatory	Number of Therapeutic Injections per Beneficiary Seen	P	S
	Average Diagnostic Procedures per Beneficiary Seen	P	S
	Average Visits per Beneficiary Seen		P
Inpatient	Percent Discharges with Vague Diagnoses	P	
	Percent Discharges with Complications	P	
	Discharges per 100 Visits	P	
	Average Length of Stay— Special Interest Procedures	P	P
	Average Hospital Costs— Special Interest Procedures		P
	Average Length of Stay— Special Interest Diagnoses	P	P
	Average Hospital Costs— Special Interest Diagnoses		P
Supplemental information	Percent Discharges with Common Surgical Procedures		
	Percent Discharges with Special Interest Procedures		
	Percent Discharges with Special Interest Diagnoses		

P = Primary Objective
S = Secondary Objective

Table 5
SUR Quality Review Variables, Beneficiary

Variable	Objectives	
	Quality	Cost
Total Visits per Beneficiary		P
Total Expenditures (Excluding Inpatient Hospital Amounts per Beneficiary)		P
Ambulatory Care Providers Seen by Beneficiary	P	
Total Expenditures per Beneficiary		P

P = Primary Objective

Table 6
Number of Diagnostic Procedures per Beneficiary Seen, Fiscal Quarter Ending 03/31/77

REGION =   OFFICE =

DIAGNOSTIC PROCEDURES

1. 70002-76999 RADIOLOGY & ULTRASOUND
2. 05601-05761 RADIOLOGY & ULTRASOUND (NS)
3. 80003-89399 LABORATORY & PATHOLOGY
4. 05791-05921 LABORATORY & PATHOLOGY (NS)
5. 05261-05265 ELECTROCARDIOGRAPHY

REPORTING CATEGORY - GROUPS AND CLINICS

PROVIDER NUMBER AND NAME	BILLING PLAN	AVG. DIAG. PROCED./ BEN SEEN	STD. DEV.	TOTAL BEN. SEEN	TOTAL DIAGNOSTIC PROCEDURES	DIAGNOSTIC PROCEDURES				
						1	2	3	4	5
PROVIDER	A (1)	1.25	2.14	126	158	6	6	127	18	1
	B (6)	1.14	2.47	569	651	0	0	622	14	15
	C (1)	0.89	0.70	74	64	0	0	64	0	0
	D (6)	0.77	1.80	227	174	0	0	165	9	0
	E (6)	0.70	1.07	240	169	0	0	161	0	0
	F (5)	0.57	1.22	423	243	37	9	185	7	5
	G (1)	0.50	1.15	397	200	0	0	190	10	0
	H (1)	0.45	1.14	134	62	0	1	46	0	1
	I (1)	0.44	1.07	299	132	7	6	89	27	3
	J (1)	0.36	0.43	286	104	0	0	98	0	1
	K (1)	0.29	0.73	290	85	2	11	68	0	6
	L (1)	0.28	0.57	65	18	0	0	14	0	0
	M (1)	0.25	0.50	89	22	0	0	22	0	0

Category		col1	col2	Total						
N	(1)	0.24	0.52	107	26	0	7	1	0	9
O	(1)	0.18	0.59	240	42	0	0	42	0	2
P	(8)	0.10	0.41	245	0	0	0	7	0	1
Q	(1)	0.08	0.31	280	18	0	1	0	0	0
R	(1)	0.04	0.26	178	21	0	0	2	2	0
S	(1)	0.02	0.15	91	7	0	0	0	1	0
T	(1)	0.02	0.19	258	2	0	0	2	0	0
U	(1)	0.00	0.12	65	3	0	0	3	0	0
V	(1)	0.00	0.00	78	0	0	0	0	0	0
W	(6)	0.00	0.00	160	0	0	0	0	0	0
X	(1)	0.00	0.00	205	0	0	0	0	0	0
Y	(1)	0.00	0.00	69	0	0	0	0	0	0
Z	(1)	0.00	0.00	156	0	0	0	0	0	0
AA	(1)	0.00	0.00							

TOTALS FOR REPORTING CATEGORY	TOTAL PROVIDERS									
OFFICE TOTALS	27	0.41		5,486	2,212	62	51	1,939	61	75
REGION TOTALS	42	0.62		13,565	8,347	749	414	6,560	294	330
FUNDS TOTALS	293	0.70		135,603	94,165	10,556	9,001	65,540	5,909	5,144

Table 7
Average Length of Stay for Special Interest Diagnoses, Fiscal Quarter Ending 03/31/77

REGION -   OFFICE -

SPECIAL INTEREST DIAGNOSES (SID)

1. 410.0-411.9 ACUTE ISCHEMIC HEART DIS	2. 412.0-414.9 CHRONIC ISCHEMIC HEART DIS	3. 427.0-427.9 HEART FAILURE	
4. 460.0-470.9 URI & INFLUENZA	5. 480.0-486.9 PNEUMONIA	6. 489.0-496.9 BRONCH, EMPHYSEMA & ASTHMA	
7. 516.0-517.9 PNEUMOCONIOSIS & CHRON FIBR	8. 140.0-209.9 ALL MALIGNANT NEOPLASMS	9. 430.0-438.9 CEREBROVASCULAR DISEASE	
10. 400.0-405.9 HYPERTENSIVE DISEASE	11. 540.0-543.9 APPENDICITIS	12. 574.0-575.9 CHOLELITHIASIS & CHOLECYST	
13. 001.0-009.9 ENTERITIS & DYSENTRY	14. 531.0-534.9 ULCER OF UPPER GI	15. 250.0-250.9 DIABETES MELLITUS	
16. 626.0-627.9 MENSTRUAL & MENO DISORDERS	17. 711.0-715.9 ARTHRITIS (EXC ACUTE)	18. 380.0-389.9 DISEASE OF EAR & MASTOID	
19. 306.0-312.9 NONPHYS PSYCH, NEUROSIS ETC	20. 313.0-314.9 DRUG DEPENDENCE & ALCOHOLISM		

REPORTING CATEGORY - SHORT TERM HOSPITAL

AVG. LOS BY SID CATEGORY

PROVIDER NUMBER AND NAME	BILLING PLAN	TOTAL SID DISCHARGES	1 / 10 / 19	2 / 11 / 20	3 / 12	4 / 13	5 / 14	6 / 15	7 / 16	8 / 17	9 / 18
HOSPITAL A	(1)	25	0.0 / 0.0 / 5.0	0.0 / 0.0 / 5.0	0.0 / 0.0	0.0 / 0.0	0.0 / 0.0	0.0 / 14.0	0.0 / 0.0	4.8 / 0.0	29.0 / 2.5
HOSPITAL B	(1)	24	5.0 / 0.0	0.0 / 0.0	0.0 / 0.0	3.0 / 3.0	0.0 / 0.0	0.0 / 0.0	0.0 / 0.0	0.0 / 0.0	0.0 / 0.0
HOSPITAL C	(3)	22	6.0 / 0.0	0.0 / 0.0	5.0 / 0.0	6.3 / 3.0	0.0 / 0.0	9.5 / 4.7	0.0 / 3.5	0.0 / 0.0	0.0 / 12.0
HOSPITAL D	(1)	24	0.0 / 5.0 / 2.0	0.0 / 8.0 / 5.0	0.0 / 0.0	3.3 / 3.0	4.0 / 0.0	6.3 / 23.7	0.0 / 5.0	3.0 / 0.0	10.0 / 0.0
HOSPITAL E	(3)	96	2.0 / 2.5 / 1.0	1.0 / 3.6 / 12.7	2.0 / 6.3	5.1 / 2.5	5.6 / 5.3	5.0 / 12.8	4.0 / 1.0	10.3 / 0.0	0.0 / 3.3
HOSPITAL F	(3)	28	3.0 / 6.3 / 4.5	0.0 / 0.0 / 0.0	0.0 / 12.5	10.3 / 4.0	3.0 / 1.0	3.0 / 8.0	4.0 / 4.0	15.7 / 23.0	0.0 / 2.0

		TOTAL PROVIDERS									
HOSPITAL G	(3)	104	9.5 4.0	11.7 9.0	7.0 9.6	1.9 6.2	5.1 4.3	4.3 7.0	0.0 4.5	6.4 7.0	11.0 7.6
HOSPITAL H	(3)	21	7.0 0.0	0.0 0.0	13.0 0.0	3.3 0.0	0.0 0.0	3.0 14.0	0.0 8.0	5.0 4.0	26.5 3.0
HOSPITAL I	(3)	59	0.0 0.0	27.0 0.0	0.0 15.3	2.4 3.0	5.5 12.7	7.9 7.0	0.0 2.0	10.5 0.0	0.0 3.5
HOSPITAL J	(3)	65	14.0 0.0	0.0 0.0	0.0 9.0	3.0 5.8	8.0 2.0	5.0 14.7	3.0 4.5	15.3 12.0	3.0 2.0
HOSPITAL K	(3)	20	14.0 0.0	0.0 0.0	0.0 12.0	5.0 0.0	4.0 0.0	5.3 7.0	0.0 2.0	0.0 12.0	0.0 3.0
HOSPITAL L	(3)	46	7.0 0.0	5.1 0.0	0.0 7.5	8.7 7.3	14.0 4.0	7.0 15.3	0.0 3.4	20.0 0.0	0.0 4.4
TOTALS FOR REPORTING CATEGORY			6.0 5.0	0.0							
OFFICE TOTALS		554	8.5 6.5 9.4	7.5 8.8 5.2	6.8 10.5	3.8 4.0	5.7 6.0	5.7 12.3	3.8 4.1	10.5 11.6	23.2 3.6
REGION TOTALS		1,961	7.7 6.3 10.1	6.7 7.0 5.3	9.8 8.5	3.5 4.0	5.2 8.2	5.5 11.6	4.8 3.0	9.6 9.3	15.1 2.9
FUNDS TOTALS		16,646	8.5 9.6 8.7	7.0 5.1 8.3	7.1 7.8	3.2 3.6	5.4 6.3	5.5 6.4	5.4 3.6	9.0 6.1	7.3 3.1

Table 8
Hospitalization Cost for Special Interest Diagnoses, Fiscal Quarter Ending 03/31/77

REGION -   OFFICE -

SPECIAL INTEREST DIAGNOSES (SID)

1. 410.0-411.9 ACUTE ISCHEMIC HEART DIS	2. 412.0-414.9 CHRONIC ISCHEMIC HEART DIS	3. 427.0-427.9 HEART FAILURE
4. 460.0-470.9 URI & INFLUENZA	5. 480.0-486.9 PNEUMONIA	6. 489.0-496.9 BRONCH, EMPHYSEMA & ASTHMA
7. 516.0-517.9 PNEUMOCONIOSIS & CHRON FIBR	8. 140.0-209.9 ALL MALIGNANT NEOPLASMS	9. 430.0-438.9 CEREBROVASCULAR DISEASE
10. 400.0-405.9 HYPERTENSIVE DISEASE	11. 540.0-543.9 APPENDICITIS	12. 574.0-575.9 CHOLELITHIASIS & CHOLECYST
13. 001.0-009.9 ENTERITIS & DYSENTRY	14. 531.0-534.9 ULCER OF UPPER GI	15. 250.0-250.9 DIABETES MELLITUS
16. 626.0-627.9 MENSTRUAL & MENO DISORDERS	17. 711.0-715.9 ARTHRITIS (EXC ACUTE)	18. 380.0-389.9 DISEASE OF EAR & MASTOID
19. 306.0-312.9 NONPHYS PSYCH, NEUROSIS ETC	20. 313.0-314.9 DRUG DEPENDENCE & ALCOHOLISM	

REPORTING CATEGORY - SHORT TERM HOSPITAL

PROVIDER NUMBER AND NAME	BILLING PLAN	TOT. SID DISCHAR.	AVG. HOSPITALIZATION COST BY SID CATEGORY								
			1 / 10 / 19	2 / 11 / 20	3 / 12	4 / 13	5 / 14	6 / 15	7 / 16	8 / 17	9 / 18
HOSPITAL A	(1)	25	0	0	0	0	0	0	0	348	53
			0	0	0	0	0	2,489	0	0	173
			0	0							
HOSPITAL B	(1)	24	42	0	0	0	0	0	0	0	0
			0	0	0	11	0	0	0	0	0
			0	0							
HOSPITAL C	(3)	22	0	0	0	10	0	167	0	0	0
			10	0	0	10	0	12	69	0	10
			0	0							
HOSPITAL D	(1)	24	124	1,229	0	655	502	999	0	905	718
			357	1,238	0	370	0	4,335	1,028	0	0
			0	0							
HOSPITAL E	I(3)	96	114	386	228	345	637	539	404	1,162	0
			263	1,305	683	279	474	812	114	-	351
			330	0							
HOSPITAL F	N(3)	28	903	0	1,749	1,354	396	396	503	2,048	0
			0	0	0	503	125	1,261	528	2,897	264
			598	0							

Provider		Total Providers / Count									
HOSPITAL G	(3)	104	1,185	1,538	904	248	644	578	0	944	1,661
			514	1,159	1,297	603	393	1,057	592	1,057	904
HOSPITAL H	(3)	21	1,026	0	1,590	398	0	367	0	611	616
			0	3,303	0	0	0	1,715	131	489	367
HOSPITAL I	(3)	59	2,202	489	0	363	872	1,233	0	1,649	0
			0	944	2,354	478	2,023	1,043	323	0	510
HOSPITAL J	(3)	65	1,025	850	0	541	1,443	902	469	2,758	541
			1,132	918	1,623	1,017	360	2,582	812	2,165	360
			2,105	1,173							
			1,287	0							
			2,374								
HOSPITAL K	(3)	20	1,852	0	0	396	551	724	264	0	0
			1,852	1,289	1,719	0	0	926	1,567	396	
			925	925							
			0	788							
			1,296	810							
HOSPITAL L	(3)	46	1,296	810	0	1,404	2,268	1,134	0	3,240	0
			810	0	1,215	1,106	648	2,160	551	0	713

TOTALS FOR REPORTING CATEGORY

Category	Total Providers	Count									
OFFICE TOTALS	12	534	1,215	1,038	683	420	787	748	445	1,517	344
			845	1,186	1,522	367	804	1,741	499	1,639	416
			1,580	777							
REGION TOTALS	26	1,961	1,210	1,687	337	417	803	845	850	1,914	813
			933	1,030	1,346	441	1,161	1,744	449	1,263	486
			1,346	755							
FUNDS TOTALS	169	16,646	1,173	1,246	1,064	322	709	698	688	1,431	805
			486	834	1,225	434	920	951	595	894	389
			982	986							

Tables 6 through 8 show actual data. Chapter 14 of this volume, by Bicknell and Kelch, notes some strategies for using such data.

Assessing the UMWA System

Does a managed, self-insured system provide cost savings, quality controls, and beneficiary satisfaction? From the UMWA Funds' experience, I believe that such a system is clearly cost effective. Analyses done from our automated claims system for the first six months of 1977 show that we are providing significant levels of medical care to our beneficiaries at costs that are very reasonable in comparison with other plans (see table 9).

Table 9
Comparison of UMWA Funds Expenditures with Other Health Benefit Programs

Program	Cost per Beneficiary
Total National Expenditures, 1976[a]	$551
Federal Employee Benefit Plan[b] Blue Cross–Blue Shield High Option (as of January 1977)	675.
National Medicaid, 1976[c]	616.
UMWA Funds, 1977 (includes all dollars spent for all beneficiaries before Medicare reimbursement)	360.

	Cost per cardholder (or policyholder)
General Motors Health Benefits Program, BC-BS of Michigan, 1976[d]	$1,199
UMWA Funds, 1976 (includes all dollars spent for all beneficiaries before Medicare reimbursement)	984

[a]Figure calculated by dividing total United States health care expenditures for 1976 by total United States population for 1976.
[b]Figure calculated by taking BC-BS individual high-option annual premium, reduced by 7 percent for administrative costs and contributions to reserves.
[c]DHEW, SRS, Medical Services Administration, *Medicaid FY 1978–1982*, September 1976, p. 2.
[d]GM's 1976 premium for UAW employees (without the dental care benefit) was $107.40 per month. Cost per cardholder is the annual premium reduced by 7 percent for administrative expenses.
Source of data: Tom Stretline, UAW, GM Div.

Additional savings would be possible through analyses of data on high-cost beneficiaries and high-cost providers. We have found that 44 percent of our expenditures are for hospital care, and (based on claims data for 30 percent of the covered population) that 7.4 percent of cardholders using care accounted for 41.5 percent of expenditures during the first six months of 1977. Hospitalization and the costs associated with treatment of acute and serious illness accounted for nearly 80 percent of the funds' total expenditures while preventive, rehabilitative, and other "nonacute" illness treatment procedures accounted for less than 2 percent. Were similar data presented in the corporate world in a non-health benefit context, I am reasonably sure it would attract considerable management attention. I believe that a heavy management effort could change the mix and reduce the cost.

The quality issue and the question of beneficiary satisfaction are much more difficult to address with any sense of optimism. The prevailing attitude in American health care today focuses on process and not outcome. The emphasis is care not cure, perhaps appropriately because of the increasing chronicity of our population's illnesses. Nonetheless, it frustrates quality assessment. SUR represents a fine beginning, but unless the physician/provider is interested in engaging on that attitudinal issue, quality control is going to remain elusive.

Beneficiary satisfaction may present even greater problems than quality controls. Beneficiaries want a health benefit that has three characteristics: freedom of choice; prompt payment, preferably through assigned claims; and no rejected claims. All three run counter to a managerially effective claims payment mechanism and a managed health system. You need some controls over market (and thus limits on freedom of choice); you need time to analyze claims carefully and investigate excessive charges; and, regrettably, you must reject some claims. There are solutions to this conflict involving both educational and incentive programs. Savings must be shared with participants, either directly or through improved benefits.

The UMWA Funds' health program data system as described above was developed over a two-year period from 1975 to 1977. The program was fully implemented in July 1977. For the most part, claims payments were occurring on a 28- to 45-day cycle for "clean" claims and on a 60-day or greater cycle for problem claims. About 12 percent of claims were rejected, largely because the beneficiary was not eligible on the date of service.

The Future of the Funds' Health Program

The 1978 National Bituminous Coal Wage Agreement ratified on March 24, 1978, after the longest coal strike in this nation's history (110 days) removed from the funds the responsibility for administering the health benefits for working miners and those recently retired. Of the more than 800,000 beneficiaries served by the funds in 1977, more than 580,000 were transferred to private health insurance carriers by June 1, 1978. The remaining 220,000, (130,000 of these covered by Medicare) remain our responsibility. The contract further eliminated the concept of a participating provider, mail-out drugs, and prepayments (for providers other than HMOs). It is unlikely that any semblance of a management data system can be maintained. The regional system is being reduced from twenty offices to eight, and these will have no responsibility for health.

The reasons for these changes are complex, but it is fair to say that beneficiary dissatisfaction with a managed system played at least a small role. A much larger factor was the companies' desire to gain control over what they viewed as their fringe benefit program.

Despite these changes, those associated with the development of this system believe that it offers a sound, workable approach to a managed health benefits package.

United Storeworkers Security Plan

William Michelson and Eleanor J. Tilson

13

Trade unions have an important stake, both economically and socially, in making health systems more equitable and efficient. All unions negotiate for health benefits of one kind or another and therefore become involved in the health problems of their memberships. Our most direct stake is that the higher costs of health must often be paid at the expense of higher wages. Relatively few union health funds have gone the route of self-insurance. We feel that this is unfortunate because self-insurance, when properly administered, can be the most effective means of providing quality care and assuring cost control.

Health Benefits Package

The United Storeworkers Union represents some 12,000 workers in major department stores in New York City and in a number of suburban branches. We provide full family coverage for a broad range of benefits, as well as covering our 1,500 retired members. In all, our Welfare Plan provides for the health care needs of some 30,000 persons. Benefits include hospitalization, medical, disability, sick leave days, dental, optical, drug, and life insurance.

The plan is totally self-insured. It is financed by employer payments which now equal 7 percent of payroll. All the monies received by the plan represent portions of previously negotiated wage increases set aside during collective bargaining by our members for the purposes of financing their health care services. We view our plan as a health cooperative and its monies as our members' monies. This concept is constantly brought to the attention of our members at meetings, in reports, in our newspapers, and in discussions.

Quality and Cost Control

We constantly educate our members to understand that the plan is a health instrument designed to get the maximum dollar value and the maximum quality care. Accordingly, we set up a panel of doctors, specialists in every field, whose qualifications we very carefully reviewed. We made certain that the doctors were board-certified in their specialties and that their hospital affiliations were with the best voluntary hospitals. The doctors on the panel all agree to accept a lower fee than they normally would receive. Evidence of the membership's confidence in what the union has provided and recommends is their high utilization of panel doctors.

Because we examine and pay all our claims, we are constantly reviewing the quality and quantity of medical services used. Together with the plan's medical adviser, we have no hesitancy in intervening when we feel there is a question as to the quality of care. Doctors are regularly informed if their performance does not measure up and are dropped from the panel whenever necessary.

In addition, we have negotiated with almost all the hospitals in New York a rate that closely approximates the Blue Cross rate. Since we pay all our own bills, we are able to scrutinize each and every claim, check lengths of stay, coordinate benefits wherever there is double coverage. When our members are in the hospital we stay in close contact with them through a team of voluntary retirees who regularly visit them and serve as ombudsmen. They report on the level of care our members are receiving and on any problems that exist where we can be of help. In many instances we have been able to reduce a hospital stay by several days through this direct communication and intervention. Where it is feasible, we arrange for home care services at a charge far lower than that of a longer hospital stay.

In the early 1970s, when we became convinced that much unnecessary surgery was being performed in this country, we set up a mandatory second surgical opinion program in conjunction with surgeons at Cornell Medical School. Whenever a member of our union is told by a surgeon that surgery is necessary, he or she is required to go for a second opinion. There have been 1,500 such mandatory second opinion consultations and 290 of our members

Table 1
Storeworkers Security Plan Comparative Statements of Operations, Fiscal Years 1976, 1977, 1978

	1978	1977	1976
Income			
Employers' contributions	$3,963,987	$3,863,651	$3,418,555
Members' direct payments	160,398	151,397	125,421
Net income from investments	265,578	278,915	205,084
Total Income	$4,389,963	$4,293,963	$3,749,060
Deduct: Benefits and Expenses			
Accident and sickness benefits	$ 739,654	$ 745,586	$ 743,145
Hospitalization benefits	1,024,233	1,020,116	992,322
Health insurance plan premiums	169,426	218,882	166,081
Medical-surgical benefits			
(fee for service)	541,721	532,125	543,541
Pre-surgical screening	20,205	18,017	19,956
Death benefits	142,827	183,126	127,484
Sick leave benefits	341,997	336,226	299,451
Cash withdrawals—death benefits	834	561	442
Medicare	226,181	183,286	194,050
Pharmacy benefits	315,069	298,551	281,183
Podiatry benefits	6,951	7,250	8,240
Optical benefits	40,251	33,430	36,799
Diagnostic benefits	20,661	26,786	24,433
Retirees' pharmacy benefits	25,170	20,640	21,450
Dental benefits	81,365	90,946	77,622
Hypertension program	47,380	30,835	11,856
Total Benefits	$3,743,925	$3,746,363	$3,548,055
Storeworkers Security Plan			
administrative fund	462,196	440,704	400,276
General expenses	25,938	22,993	20,408
Total benefits and expenses	$4,232,059	$4,210,060	$3,968,739
Net increase (decrease) in accumulated			
reserves for the year	$ 157,904	$ 83,903	$ 219,679)
Net increase (decrease) in market			
Values for the year	$ (213,548)	$ 148,547	$ 272,707
Comparative Income (Accrual Basis)			
Employer contributions	$4,046,124	$3,858,159	$3,429,467
Other income	425,976	430,312	330,505
Total Income	$4,472,100	$4,288,471	$3,759,972

declined surgery as a result. Our statistics show that above and beyond the 20 percent drop in hospital admissions for surgery that our records reveal, we are seeing an additional 12 percent decrease in hospital admissions for surgery and we are convinced it is due to our program. The savings to the plan resulting from the second opinion come close to $1 million.

Another program we launched with the help of the Cornell Medical School is a work site testing and treatment program for hypertension. We enlisted the support of each of the major stores we have under contract to permit testing on their premises. Some 76 percent of our membership participated in the testing. Those who were found to be hypertensive were offered treatment either at the work site or as close to it as possible. The two major treatment locations are the two local union headquarters across the street from the two major department stores under contract; four other treatment centers are located on the employers' premises. Treatment is under the supervision of a doctor, but ongoing care—dispensing medication, checking blood pressure, checking weight, and so forth—is performed by a nurse therapist who sees the patients regularly. Participants receive a thorough physical examination by the doctor twice a year. Over 500 members are now receiving treatment at the program's six locations.

Its effectiveness is evident from the statistics we keep and monitor regularly. During its four years of existence, this program has retained more participants and lowered their blood pressure to normal levels than has any other hypertension program in this country. There has also been a decrease in sick days, hospital days, and other medically related costs for this group of members as compared with a group of members who chose not to come into the program but whom we are monitoring. We expect that the real dollar saving will first be perceived after a longer period of time.

Another effort that has proven cost effective is a disability evaluation program. A member who is out on a disability for longer than what has been medically determined as a normal length of stay for his or her condition is sent for an evaluation. In some instance, the evaluation has revealed a more serious ailment than that reported in the initial doctor's disability claims information. Overall, however, length of stay per disability for our members has gone down over the past three to four years to an average of thirty-three days—well below the national average.

It is clear to us that our ability to control our health care costs, to control quality, and to launch effective health programs is a result of self-insurance: we could not have achieved it through a third-party insurer. By maintaining the health records of our members and then monitoring both services and charges, we have been able to set up innovative health care and prevention programs that would meet members' needs in a cost-effective way. Our statement of operations for the past several years has shown this most dramatically, and the Board of Trustees of our Health Fund has demonstrated their wholehearted support for what we have done.

AN ACTION PLAN

William J. Bicknell

Industry and Insurer Interventions to Control the Costs of Health Benefits

William J. Bicknell and Brant Kelch

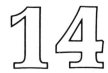

The costs of employee health benefits are growing out of proportion to the scope of the benefit and often faster than the balance of the compensation package. Even though health benefit costs are pretax dollars, they are now such a significant percentage of total compensation costs that corporate management must critically examine them and determine whether there are better ways to purchase a given level of benefit.

This paper is designed to assist corporate management in answering several questions critical to effective cost containment of the health benefit package:

What role can insurance carriers play?

Is a fully self-insured and self-administered plan a reasonable option?

What are the likely consequences and payoffs of various specific company-initiated interventions in the personal health care delivery system?

Caveats and Context

The individual interventions suggested in this chapter are for the most part neither new nor untried. However, the use of a broad range of intervention strategies within a company to contain the cost of the health care benefit is unusual and requires close collaboration between legal counsel and corporate health and benefit staffs.

This chapter alludes to legal aspects of intervention strategies. Confidentiality, antitrust and liability issues must be faced squarely and are discussed in more detail in Chapter 15, by John Blum. Even though a company's total program could readily be interpreted as fostering competition, consumer choice, and improving the market, there is without question a need to determine for each type of intervention and for patterns of intervention the risk of a law suit, its potential seriousness, the risk of adverse judgment, and the steps required to minimize unfavorable decisions.

This chapter does not discuss in detail company-sponsored health monitoring and services, whether required by OSHA (for example, exposure level monitoring, employee screening) or volitional on the part of the company (alcoholism programs, counseling for employees with family problems, employee health education and primary care clinics). However, all are compatible with and, when appropriate, easily integrated into any of the approaches discussed in this paper.

Our consideration of interventions takes place in a context of growing public and private concern over the cost of medical care—understandable concerns when one realizes that:

> Total national health expenditures have increased from $12 billion in 1960 to $160.6 billion in 1977.[1]
>
> Per capita health expenditures over the same period have increased almost tenfold, from $78 to $730.[2]
>
> The cost of a typical day in a hospital in 1977 was more than twelve[3] times what it was in 1950.[4]
>
> Physician fees increased by 50 percent more than other consumer prices in 1977.[5]
>
> Most of the increase in health care costs is attributable not to quality improvement nor increased use of services but to a health care inflation rate that has significantly outpaced the consumer price index for all items and services.[6]

The results are reflected in the growth of health expenditures as a percentage of gross national product (GNP), from 4.6 percent in 1950 to 8.8 percent in 1977.[7] At the present rate of increase, 9.6 percent of GNP will be devoted to health in 1982.[8]

Increased productivity and automation have dramatically reduced employment opportunities in the once labor-intensive farm and factory relative to the size of the population. This has occurred while the American population has been growing and expectations have been rising for well-compensated, socially valued employment. These factors are among the subtle but powerful and pervasive driving forces promoting increases in the more labor-intensive service sector of the economy. Health—more precisely, medical care—is in the service sector. Medical care is readily, although erroneously, equated with health,[9] and often valued beyond its apparent worth. This makes it yet easier for public and private expenditures to grow with few restraints.

There are other factors increasing cost: technology, whether appropriate or inappropriate and whatever its value, is always costly; an oversupply of physicians and hospital beds; excessive prescribing and use of medical services; and, perhaps most important, a gradual and fundamental change in one basic check on excess—the reimbursement mechanism. In the "good old days" when insurance coverage was limited or absent and Medicare and Medicaid were undreamed of cornucopias, both doctor and patient knew that an office visit or a hospital stay would cost the patient money out of pocket. In 1935, 83 percent of the health care expenditures were paid directly by the patient.[10] The doctor knew that his decisions in large measure had to be affordable to his patients. There is no question that this system had drawbacks, among them financial barriers to access, the fostering of a dual standard of care with grossly inadequate care for very low income groups and minorities, and, on occasion, the substitution of not only less costly but far less desirable care. However, the important point that has been largely lost in today's reimbursement climate is straightforward: services were exchanged for money and the money was usually out of pocket—a real and immediate expense felt by the patient and appreciated by the practitioner.

Since 1935, direct payment as a proportion of total payment for health care has decreased by 60 percent.[11] While the payment basis—a fee for a specific service—is unchanged, payment and service have been largely uncoupled in the minds of patient and doctor, their connection eroded to the vanishing point by third-party payments. The result is akin to putting a child in the candy store with a good fairy paying the bill. Neither the merchant nor the customer can be expected to show much restraint. This is precisely the case in medical markets. Neither patients nor physicians have incentives for restraint because the third-party good fairy pays, and pays, and pays.

Only slowly are we beginning to realize that somebody has to pay the good fairy. And, except in the case of the very poor and the elderly, that somebody has become, in large measure, industry. This is a most unfortunate position. No sound businessman would give his other suppliers or brokers blank checks. But in health care, industry and, to a lesser extent, government do just that. Purchase decisions by patient and doctor, and payment decisions by third parties are totally out of the control of a major ultimate payer—industry. This is an obvious invitation to excess. Can this be changed? Yes, but with difficulty. Is it worth changing? Yes.

Why Get Involved?

Why should industry get involved in anything other than paying for an agreed-upon benefit package? After all, some say, we at XYZ Industries have enough problems taking care of our own business.

There are several reasons for involvement:

- If the health business doesn't become more industry's business, then it will become ever more the government's business. The result is predictable: higher taxes without commensurate improvement in the value of the services received, and increased involvement of government in yet another portion of the private sector.

- There is money to be saved—a significant sum of money. Textron, Inc., through a surgical cost claims control program for 36,000 employees, has, with its carrier, Aetna Life & Casualty, saved an estimated $430,000 to $630,000 annually.[12]

- While saving money, industry can influence the medical care delivery system to deliver a better product at a fairer price. This is good for employee, employer, and the country as a whole. Industry can thus demonstrate private sector problem-solving capabilities applied effectively to broad social issues.

But why bother when national health insurance may be just around the corner? No one should count on national health insurance to solve his problems. For one thing, it's been around the corner for a couple of decades. Second, and of greater importance, the system of care and the pattern of payment that exists at the time national health insurance is instituted will be the system of care and pattern of payment we as taxpayers will be forced to finance in perpetuity. Industry will have far less chance to influence the system then than it has now, even though its obligation to pay for nationally financed health care through the tax system can reasonably be expected to grow and grow and grow.

In fiscal 1967 government expenditures for health care, including Medicare and Medicaid (enacted the previous year), totaled approximately $12.5 billion; by fiscal 1976 they had increased to an estimated $48.4 billion.[13] Even at this level, government expenditures represent only 40.2 percent[14] of total personal health care expenditures—national health insurance could dwarf this figure. Industry's stake, if only as taxpayer, is clearly enormous.

Conditions for Successful Intervention

Intervention is used here to mean actions taken to ensure the efficient delivery of health services at an optimal level of quality. For such actions to be acceptable, services as perceived by consumers must be at least as good as, if not better than, those available in an unconstrained market where the consumer can shop with little if any fiscal or program restraint.

In the area of cost containment and quality improvement, employer, employee, and society all stand to benefit if intervention is sustained and effective. However, there are at present few if any industries and surprisingly few third-party payers that are *effectively* engaged in activities that either contain costs or enhance quality. This weakness on the part of carriers is a fundamental flaw in the United States reimbursement mechanism. Can carriers do more and better? Can industry stimulate carriers to be more effective, or should industry bypass carriers and intervene directly with doctors, hospitals, employees and their families, as well as planning and regulatory agencies? These are some of the fundamental issues set forth in previous chapters of this volume.

Intervening with providers, planning and regulatory agencies, and consumers is active involvement. The difference between what is going on today and what must go on tomorrow if costs are to be contained is involvement and intervention. Industry must become, either directly or through its agents (the carriers), an informed and concerned purchaser of services rather than merely a passive payer of bills.

For intervention to succeed the following ten conditions must be met:

- Quality must be preserved or enhanced.
- Consumer satisfaction must be maintained or increased.
- Savings in benefit expenditures must exceed the direct cost of intervention over a period of years. To expect instant savings is usually unrealistic.
- Savings in excess of intervention costs must be directly or indirectly shared with employees.
- Selection should be made among physicians and hospitals on grounds of cost, need, consumer satisfaction, quality, and administrative compliance.
- Data must be readily and systematically available for assessing problems and progress.
- Utilization and cost objectives must be specific, well-conceived, and achievable.
- Top management must be committed to the objectives and prepared to withstand articulate and persistent resistance from providers accustomed to passive purchasers of services.
- To the extent used, carriers must willingly and formally agree to intervene and to conform to industry-specified performance goals.
- Ultimately, firms should develop mechanisms for collaborating with other employers in the purchase of services and for coordination between themselves and the regulatory and planning agencies in a given medical trade area.

It is doubtful that there is any other item in company budgets that is less well-understood than health care, yet costs as much, is so much under the control of vendors (physicians and hospitals), and so little in control of the consumers (employees) or the payer (industry). When purchasing pencils, raw materials, or services, no one would consider it good business practice to accept all suppliers on their terms and at their asking price. Rather, requirements are defined and purchases made from a limited number of vendors who are consistently able to deliver a product or service of acceptable quality and needed quantity at a price that is affordable and in time to meet the purchaser's needs. These accepted business practices are largely suspended in the health benefit area.

Granted, health is not the primary business of most industrial firms. It is different, and making informed choices in the purchase of health services takes some expertise. The first questions a firm must ask are: Are health benefit expenditures large enough and growing fast enough to be of concern to management? What can we do? How can the firm organize to do it? The first question can be answered only in the context of a particular business. But given the overall cost figures for health services noted above, the answer in most cases is at least a qualified yes. The balance of this chapter is directed toward answering questions two and three. But neither can be addressed without first developing a solid base of facts from which the purchaser of health care services can make informed policy choices.

Data Gathering: A Necessary Step

A prerequisite to any meaningful effort at benefit management and health system intervention is data that answer the fundamental question: Who gets what services, where, delivered by whom, at what cost, and how do these patterns of utilization and cost compare with other similar populations receiving services through various delivery mechanisms?

Data Requirements

Illustrative data requirements are displayed in tables 1 through 9 in the appendix to this chapter (pp. 153–161).

Expenditure Data

What is the firm spending on health care by class: inpatient hospital; outpatient hospital; physician; drugs; nursing home; home health; durable medical equipment; etc.? How do these expenditures compare with other firms offering similar benefits (in aggregate; per capita; and as a percentage of total health care benefit expenditures)? At what rate are these expenditures changing? Table 1 provides some of these measures for specified programs. Variations in benefits and beneficiary demographics among the various programs should be investigated before making comparisons.

Population Data

Age and sex are key determinants of utilization. In general, the older the adult population and the more females, the greater the use of medical care (tables 2 and 3). To illustrate the form such data can take, table 4 presents actual United Mine Workers of America (UMWA) Health and Retirement Funds' population data as of January 1976. Although the funds' beneficiaries reside in forty-nine states plus a number of foreign countries, detailed analysis determined that 89.2 percent of total cardholders reside in 147 counties within seven states. Table 5 is a finer breakdown of population within the state containing the largest number of beneficiaries. Similar data can be developed by health systems agency (HSA) area, standard metropolitan statistical area (SMSA), or zip code. The numbers in aggregate and by major medical trade areas and as a percentage of total population (both beneficiary and total general) provide a quick overview of where leverage and/or potential savings exist and suggest priorities for initiating intervention measures.

Utilization Data

Level of utilization by type of service is important, as is some indication of how the firm is doing compared with others. For example, table 6 compares the UMWA funds' beneficiary utilization of medical care with certain other population groups. Such data, age-, sex-, and service-specific, are critical for deciding where problems exist and where the greatest potential payoff may be expected as a result of intervention. Note the variations by region in the funds' utilization despite identical benefit structures and management. Equally important but not shown here is hospital outpatient utilization data.

Resource Data

The supply and distribution of health manpower and facilities affect utilization and cost. Table 7 documents that the supply of physicians and acute hospital beds varies considerably through the United States. Knowledge of medical geography—what providers are where—is the basis for choosing among a variety of specific interventions, such as negotiating with individual providers, stimulating individual practice association HMOs, coordinating with other firms or industries, becoming a force at planning agency meetings, actively supporting enrollment in existing HMOs, or opposing construction of additional facilities. One good source of this kind of information is the National Center for Health Statistics of the U.S. Department of Health, Education, and Welfare. Table 8 is indicative of the wealth of data available through the center.

Individual Hospital and Physician Profiles

These help answer the questions of who provides most of the firm's health services, how, and at what costs. Although a firm's aggregate population, even broken down by geographic area, may be only a small percentage of the total population in that area, its employees and dependents may represent a significant share of the business of certain specific providers. For example, although the UMWA funds' beneficiary population residing in Kentucky is only about 3 percent of the total state population, 43 percent of days of care provided by McDowell Hospital in Floyd County, Kentucky, were for funds' patients. Obviously, being payer for this large a share of a provider's market represents influence.

Individual provider profiles also help in defining reasonable patterns of practice and identifying "outliers." Evidence that some providers may be flagrant abusers sets the stage for provider-specific interventions. Types of data that are essential to identifying appropriate interventions include, for hospitals:

- Size, type, number of beds, type of ownership
- Admissions, length of stay (service-specific) for all patients and your patients
- Total dollars and your percentage of total dollars
- Cost indices (per diems, ancillaries, average total expenditure per day and per admission)
- Rank-ordered discharge diagnoses (fifteen most common)
- Procedures and diagnoses of special interest; for example Caesarean sections and normal deliveries, tonsillectomy and adenoidectomy, open heart surgery, gallbladder, hysterectomy, hernia, acute myocardial infarction.

The corresponding items for physicians are:

- General practitioners and specialists by type
- Age, board-eligible, board-certified
- Visits per year and expenditures per year for your population
- Hospital admissions by physician, number and type
- Cost per visit; frequency of visits
- Ancillary procedures per visit

Patient-Specific Data and Patient Profiles

Concerns about confidentiality may lead industry to severely limit the collection of data on specific diagnoses and procedures for individual patients. Further, physician sensitivity can blunt data collection efforts unless physicians are approached slowly and with great care.

However, patient profiles are valuable as they allow identification and analysis of high and low users and nonusers of health services. The service patterns of both high and low users may be particularly important as the basis for understanding individual patient choices and for educating employees and families on how to use the delivery system appropriately, what to do for themselves, when to go for help, and how to make an informed choice of where to go. Complex and costly cases can be identified, profiled, and used as case examples to highlight weaknesses and inadequacies in the delivery system.

Some Data Strategies

Approaching Providers

Table 9, consisting of actual data from the UMWA funds' Surveillance and Utilization Review (SUR) System, demonstrates the wide variations possible for one illustrative procedure—cholecystectomy (gallbladder removal)—in average length of stay and average hospital cost on both a per case and a per day basis at given hospitals in the same medical trade area. The variations are substantial. If an analysis of patient-specific profiles reveals that age, sex, and complicating factors do not account for the variations, the firm can and should question the hospitals and physicians: Why is the average length of stay 7.6 days longer at hospital A than hospital E? Why is the cost per day at hospital C approximately 60 percent higher than at hospital E?

The tone taken in discussions with providers can be, "We care about our employees and their families and we will share our experience with you (hospital or physician) so that you can learn of our concerns and work with us in understanding our data and seeking to improve the efficiency and quality of service delivery." It is almost always true, but often overlooked or even disputed, that quality and efficiency go hand in hand; it is good management and politics to link quality and efficiency in discussions with providers.

Developing Basic Reporting Requirements

An initial national step that would be extraordinarily useful is for several firms or industries to develop together a basic health benefits data reporting requirement. This would specify the minimum data set and reporting procedures that a benefit program manager could reasonably expect of his carrier or require of his own in-house program. Not only would the data themselves be useful, as touched upon in Chapter 4, but as soon as carriers realize their performance is being closely scrutinized, they will be stimulated to think ahead and develop intervention actions aimed at cost containment and at improving their own competitive positions in the health insurance market. Thus, if enough clients merely ask the right questions, a favorable impact on cost can be anticipated. This uniform reporting system would have the additional benefit of allowing valid comparisons to be made between various carriers and employee groups.

Taking Action

The first steps toward taking action are deciding what to do and how to organize to do it. Looking first at what to do, decisions must be made concerning five components of health benefits plan management: managing cash flow; choosing among administrative mechanisms; structuring the benefit package; managing the benefit package; and intervening in the health delivery system.

Managing Cash Flow

If cash flow management has not yet been fully considered in the area of health benefits, a business may readily achieve some cost savings in that area. Carriers may not always suggest a cash flow management plan that is optimal from the purchaser's point of view. Indeed, in recent discussions with insurers, the UMWA Health and Retirement Funds found several whose suggested method of payment maximized the *carrier's* cash flow advantage over and above anything reasonably required for risk associated with potential business. Simply stated, when agreeing to the timing of premium payments, purchasers should consider the time value of money as much as the time when the carrier will actually incur expenses on the policyholder's behalf.

Accordingly, in dealing with carriers, it is prudent to challenge their reserve accumulation requirements. This does not imply that reserves are a superfluous expense; they are the insurance industry's means of dealing with fluctuation contingencies. But what a carrier "requires" and what is sufficient to cover the contingencies resulting from your policy often differ significantly. Insist on a full explanation of the specific purpose(s) and use(s) of required reserves.

A carrier often has more flexibility in its reserve requirements than it reveals during a contract negotiation. For example, Blue Cross plans may request a firm to provide the equivalent of three months of benefit and administrative expense dollars over and above a normal premium payment sufficient to cover benefit and administrative expenses. This complies with the National Blue Cross Association standards for approval of financial responsibility for Blue Cross plans within the United States, but in truth, the standards are more easily satisfied:

> "A Plan's reserves shall be decided minimally adequate if they meet one of the three following criteria:
>
> a. They are sufficient to meet hospital and operating expenses for a period of at least three months; or
>
> b. they have been increased by the addition of at least 3 percent of gross income during the preceding twelve month period; or
>
> c. they will be increased or not drastically reduced during the forthcoming twelve month period, based upon projection of next year's operations."[15]

Complying with criterion a could mean, for every $1 million expended on employee benefit utilization and Blue Cross administrative expenses, an additional $250,000 is provided for carrier use. At 6 percent interest, this represents $15,000 the first year of the contract. Complying with criterion c, on the other hand, could mean that none of the $250,000 is needed.

The policyholder can determine the actual value of the money provided to or requested by a carrier through a number of measures: cost of borrowing funds; cost of issuing various types of securities; rate of return on funds invested in the money market; rate of return on capital invested in the firm's business; and/or rate of return on funds invested in other markets. (However, restrictions on carriers' reserve investments may lower the interest they can actually earn.) Further, some states have statutory reserve requirements. These requirements vary widely from state to state both in the basis (percentage of premium income, x months of incurred expenses, fixed amount, etc.) and dollar levels (0 to tens of millions.) Occasionally, maximum reserve levels as well as minimums are established. It is obviously prudent for a policyholder to investigate such requirements. But regardless of carrier or even state requirements, purchasers should give serious consideration to insisting on an interest credit at competitive rates for any money provided that is held by the carrier in any type of reserve account.

Choosing Among Administrative Mechanisms

The range of possibilities for administering the benefit package covers a spectrum from fully insured and administered by a carrier to fully self-insured and self-administered (exhibit 1). Although the advantages, in terms of program control, of greater involvement in the payment and administration of health benefits are substantial, the primary factor in selecting a structure is usually cost.

Regardless of the structure chosen, claim expenses obviously remain. (Actions that can be taken to contain these costs are discussed later.) However, the choice of structure determines whether one incurs certain costs associated with the administration of the health benefits program, specifically: reserve requirements, risk and profit charges, and taxes.

The importance of minimizing reserve requirements or assuring adequate earnings has been addressed above in the section on cash flow management. Some level of reserves is usually required by state law and/or regulations for the fully insured, stop-loss, and minimum premium type of contracts, although these levels vary widely from state to state and from carrier to carrier. Under administrative services only (ASO) contracts, the carrier's reserve requirements may be avoided entirely if the employer assumes full liability for all claims incurred before the ASO contract termination date. If the employer does not choose to accept full liability, the reserve requirements may be determined by establishing a once-a-year cut-off date and tracking the dollar amount of claims paid subsequent to, but incurred prior to, termination of the carrier contract. Carriers also can use a sequential series of cut-off dates to approximate the liability at any point in time. Because provider billing practices and utilization of services are somewhat subject to seasonal fluctuations, the expected liability varies by the time of year the contract is terminated. The choice of approach is usually dependent upon the firm's rights to terminate the contract. If it can be terminated without cause at any time with x days notice, the sequential method is more appropriate, since it considers seasonal variations in benefit expenditures. If the contract is to run for a set period of time unless sufficient grounds for termination are experienced, the annual run-off may be satisfactory. Increasingly, minimum premium contracts are used similarly to reduce reserve requirements by shifting liability from the insurer to the employer. Under self-administered and self-insured plans, the employer determines the need, level, and use of reserve funds. In summary, as reserve requirements increase, net costs increase. Appropriately developed ASO contracts and self-administered/self-insured plans eliminate these requirements and thereby reduce net costs.

Risk and profit charges, including commissions and other overhead costs, are highest when a fully insured structure is chosen. Even when the claim expense can be accurately determined in advance, a risk charge of 7 percent of this expense is not an unusual add-on to premiums charged. In some instances, premiums for a fully insured program have been paid that are nearly twice the actual claims expense. For example, the UMWA Health and Retirement Funds' premium payments during a recent contract year to its carrier for the health benefits plan covering employees of the Funds exceeded actual claims expense by 79 percent. Employers should always insist on a full accounting of claims expense regardless of the type of structure chosen. Knowledge of this will enable calculation of true administrative expenses, including profits, and can be used in future negotiations of premiums. In general, as one moves along the spectrum from fully-insured to self-insured, risk and profit charges decrease.

The third major cost that is in large part determined by the administrative structure is taxes. Premium taxes vary from state to state, though they are typically 2 percent of premiums. On fully insured programs, premiums are highest and therefore premium taxes are highest. Minimum premium administrative/financing structures were developed primarily to avoid premium taxes and do so in many states. Other states, in response to lost revenues, apply taxes nearly equivalent to those incurred under the fully insured option to the modified insurance and, in some cases, even the ASO structures. A self-insured/self-administered 501(c)(9) trust for health benefits is exempt from paying premium taxes. Similarly, investment earnings and capital gains on the trust funds are exempt from federal and state income taxes, which can result in significant savings. For example, each $1 million in reserves invested at 6 percent earns $60,000 annually. Corporate income taxes of 40 percent would eliminate $24,000 of these earnings, thereby increasing net costs. Reserves invested by many carriers are subject to income taxes resulting in reduced interest earnings payable back to the policyholder. In dollar terms tax savings are an important cost consideration in selecting an administrative structure. Again, fully insured is typically the most costly and self-administered/self-insured the least costly structure.

In summary, a self-insured/self-administered plan can in most cases avoid a minimum of 2 to 4 percent of the costs incurred under a fully insured structure. This makes it easy to understand why, between 1972 and 1975, Blue Cross and Blue Shield plans lost more contracts to self-insured/self-administered programs than to all commercial carriers combined. By 1976 the Blues felt that the various self-insurance and self-administration approaches could be considered, in aggregate the third largest "carrier," ranking only below the Blues and Aetna.[16] Many in the insurance industry consider it their greatest challenge for future growth.

Why the recent increase in self-insurance? There are six basic reasons:

• Corporate financial conditions are tighter.

• Premiums have increased dramatically in the past few years.

• Awareness of risk and profit charges and of reserve and premium tax considerations has increased.

• ERISA removes a major legal reason for not insuring. Section 514(b)2 states, "Neither an employee benefit plan . . . nor any trust established under such plan, shall be deemed to be an insurance company or other insurer for purposes of any law of any state purporting to regulate insurance companies, insurance contracts."

Exhibit 1
Structures for Administering Health Benefits

Structure	Description	Reserve Requirements	Risk and Profit Charges	Premium Taxes	Major Advantages
I. Fully Insured	Fixed amount paid insurer (per family unit) who assumes liability for all claims.	Generally 2–3 months requested	For a large case 0.5–0.7%[a] of premium is typical	All payments taxed	Predictable fixed expenditures (no risk)
II. Modified Insurance					
A. Minimum Premium					
1. Variation A	Employer is responsible for all claims up to a predetermined annual dollar level (usually 90% of projected claims) and the insurer pays all in excess. Insurer also commits to pay below excess, if employer does not, and be reimbursed later	Generally 2–3 months requested	Roughly 0.3–0.4%[a]	Varies by state. In some states only applied to excess coverage (top layer). In Mich., Cal., Conn. & Texas, e.g., based on all claims paid by both parties	In some states significant premium tax savings
2. Variation B	Similar to variation A but the excess is determined on a monthly basis.	Generally 2–3 months requested	Roughly 0.3–0.4%[a]	Same as variation A	Same as variation A plus cash flow advantages
B. Stop Loss	Any claims in excess of a predetermined dollar limit are the liability of the insurer and not recoverable.	Generally 2–3 months requested	Set at 150% of projected claims, typical ranges 0.25–0.3%[a]	All payments taxed	Less expensive than fully insured and prevents catastrophic losses
III. Administrative Services Only	Provides administrative services (claims processing, etc.) without insurer risk assumption. Employer self-insurers and purchases claim payment services.	If the employer assumes all liabilities after termination date, only reserve requirements are self-determined.	With appropriate termination charge regarding employer liability risk charges can be avoided	Varies by state–usually no premium tax. In some states such as Connecticut and Idaho payments are subject to tax.	Better control of cash flow reduces "retentions" through reserve requirements and in some states eliminates premium taxes.

IV. Self-Administered and Self-Insured	Employer performs administration functions without external assistance or insurance.				
A. Single and Multiple Employer Trusts	Section 501(c)9 of Internal Revenue Code permits establishment of a tax-exempt trust for payment of health benefits.	0 (self-determined if established)	0	0 (in most states) ERISA exempts such trusts from coming under state insurance law and regulation.	No risk and profit charges. Usually no premium or income taxes. No contractual reserves. Greater control over the program including cash flow.
B. Internal to Company (Employer-Provided)	Payments for benefits made directly by employer from corporate funds.	0 (self-determined if established)	0	Varies subject to state "insurance" laws and regulations.	No risk and profit charges. More subject to insurance law than 501(c)9 trusts but generally less premium taxes than other structures. Similar to trusts in control over program and cash flow but earnings are subject to income taxes where 501(c)9 trust income is not.

[a]Source: *Employee Benefit Plan Review Research Reports*, Published by Charles D. Spencer and Associates, Chicago, 1976.

- Administrative services only contracts, developed in the 1970s, allow companies unwilling to assume the administrative claims processing functions to self-insure but contract out the processing activities.

- The success of other companies has become known. For example, in December 1975 the Washington Business Group on Health surveyed its members and found that of the thirty-six members who changed to self-insurance, thirty-three indicated cost savings as a primary reason and result. This experience was described in the Council on Wage and Price Stability report of December 1976.[17]

If savings can be achieved, along with greater control through involvement, why aren't even more employers moving toward self-insurance? At least four explanations can be suggested. There may be lack of knowledge of this option or misperception that radical change is necessary. Or, employees and unions may be opposed in some cases, although if they fully understood the choices and shared in the savings, such opposition may vanish. Finally, some companies may fear catastrophic costs, even though health care experience is very predictable in a reasonably large population.

With large enough numbers there can be accurate prediction of total costs *other than* those attributable to health care inflation. No one has proven to be a successful prognosticator of price changes in the health sector. Carriers in developing premiums include a liberal allowance for inflationary trends plus a risk charge. Self-insurance results in paying no more than what inflation adds to costs. The unpredictability of inflation rates does necessitate setting aside or having access to sufficient funds to offset increased prices. In determining the advisability of self-insuring and whether the risks are significant enough to preclude the opportunities to save, one should consider the following:

1. The size of the group. A group of 500 employees is generally considered large enough to be self-insured and smooth out individual fluctuations in claim expense. Groups comprising as few as 200 heads of household have successfully self-insured. Claim fluctuations in smaller groups may be significant.

2. Sufficiency and stability of income. Is the business's income within a predictable range and sufficient to set aside funds to meet fluctuating (seasonal variations, inflation, etc.) expenses?

3. Past utilization and cost experience. Comparative data discussed earlier are necessary for this assessment.

4. Geographic concentration of beneficiaries.

5. Stability of beneficiary population.

As a guideline, with 500 to 1,000 employees or from 2,000 to 4,000 total beneficiaries, it is usually possible to predict utilization so accurately that very limited insurance or none at all may well be the best decision. This immediately moves one out of the insurance business, away from retentions, generally reducing premium taxes and risk charges, and at a minimum, into a situation that has only a modicum of insurance associated with it—either to stop-loss coverage, which may be appropriate for a smaller company with tight cash flow and a wary financial officer, or to a minimum premium variation.

As a practical matter, any large group is experience-rated because the premium each year reflects the previous year's experience. The purchaser is not buying insurance but rather is buying the administration of a benefit. The question then turns on the pros and cons of different administrative structures. There are basically four options: the Blue Cross and Blue Shield plans; the commercial carriers; data processing firms; or self-administration. A fifth option also exists: special purpose groups for administering dental, vision, and pharmacy benefits. They are conceptually similar to the "Blues" to the extent that the Blues are special purpose groups founded for the administration of hospital and physician benefits.

The three chief criteria (outlined in the box) for choosing among the options include the carrier's service capabilities, the administrative costs of the

---

ADMINISTRATIVE OPTIONS EVALUATION CRITERIA

1. Service Capabilities
    a. Contract development
    b. Development of employee health benefits description booklet
    c. Development of employee identification cards
    d. Development and furnishing of all printed forms required to administer program including enrollment cards, claim forms, etc.
    e. Actuarial and legal assistance
    f. Processing and adjudication of claims including Third Party Liability determination
    g. Provider assistance and reimbursement
    h. Beneficiary assistance
    i. Statistial reporting

2. Administrative Costs
    a. For services above
    b. Reserve and retention factors
    c. Premium taxes
    d. Profits
    e. Cash flow considerations

3. Cost Containment and Quality Improvement Potential
    a. Benefit package structure
    b. Benefit package management
    c. Systems intervention

plan, and the potential for cost containment and quality improvement through benefit package structure, benefit package management, and systems intervention. The criteria can be summarized quite simply: what services are needed and provided, and at what cost? But this leads to other questions. First, which of these services can be arranged for in-house or purchased at lower cost from others who are not insurance carriers—consultants, printing firms (for benefit descriptions, ID cards, etc.), service bureaus, time-sharing operations, and so on? Second, what is the level and quality of service? For example, the evaluation of claims processing and adjudication (payment determination) takes account not only of costs but also of speed and accuracy of payments. What percentage of claims are paid within seven days? Fourteen days? Twenty-one days? What is the average turnaround (claim received to check mailed) time for claims?

Some contractors can process 90 percent of all claims within ten days of receipt. Others may take twenty-one days or more. Speed, though, is related to the manpower and machine effort involved (which translate into dollars) as well as the complexity of the review process. The complexity is a function of various factors—(1) paying only for covered services obtained by eligible beneficiaries; (2) assuring that billed services are an accurate reflection of services rendered; (3) paying no more than necessary—all of which affect the accuracy of payment. The first is relatively easy to accomplish. The second involves the detection of fraud, which is necessary from a deterrent perspective but is at best a high-cost, measurably low-yield endeavor. The third involves claims review to determine such things as excessive charges, duplicate claims, other parties' liability (such as spouse's insurance, workmen's compensation, government programs including Medicare, crippled children, black lung, accident insurance). Its effectiveness depends on the vigor with which these sources of excess charges are pursued once identified.

All claims-processing systems have weaknesses with regard to (2) and (3). It is important for the firm to know what its dollars are buying so that it can make proper comparisons and decide which weaknesses are worth correcting. Controlling erroneous expenditures costs money. It is essential to question whether the various controls such as prior authorization requirements, utilization review, fee edits, and third-party liability screens can potentially save as much as they cost. This is a major consideration in the third criterion governing the choice of insurance arrangement—potential for cost containment and quality improvement.

In selecting an option, all costs need to be included: benefit claims expenditures; administrative charges, including cost of services provided; premium taxes; reserve and other retention requirements, including profits. Some bidders for the contract will contend that their reimbursement arrangements with providers will save x percent of benefit expenditures. All such contentions require thorough investigation as they may be significantly overstated.

Administrative costs range from perhaps slightly less than 3 percent to 10 or more percent of total costs. Lower than 3 percent is difficult to obtain, and over 8 or 9 percent should be viewed with concern. Obviously, one percentage point can make a big difference—$100,000 on every $10 million dollars worth of claims. And if, as some say, savings on self-insurance and self-administration over an ASO arrangement may be several percentage points, the savings are very substantial, particularly if consistently realized over a period of years.

Sound reasons exist for considering self-administration. They include:

Better control over determination of eligibility

Control over all decisions regarding claims interpretation

Easier access for employees to personnel handling claims

Ability to identify those who overutilize services

Capability to design a plan specific to your own needs

Immediate savings from reducing or escaping the carrier's expenses passed on to employers of advertising, lobbying, public relations activities, and so on

Elimination of reserve requirements and expanded opportunities for investment

Reduction or elimination (usually) of state premium taxes

Elimination of profits and commissions paid to brokers and contractors

Tax exemption of investment earnings if a 501(c)(9) trust is established for administering benefits

Cash flow advantages through full use of money until checks are cashed, rather than mailed

Potential for better management and employee understanding of the costs of health care

Opportunity to affect the delivery system directly rather than pressuring middlemen

Potential to use company financial expertise to improve the efficiency of the delivery system

The oft-cited need for a third-party buffer to turn down claims is now less valid. In specifically requiring that all employee benefit plans provide "a full and fair review" of all claims denied by a carrier or contractors, ERISA's section 503 gives employers final authority and responsibility. Still, many organizations will deem it inadvisable, for one reason or another, to switch to self-administration. Such a decision does not preclude opportunities for improving the health care system and containing costs. It is possible, for instance, to foster competition among contractors. Carriers, the Blues, and even data processing companies are able to provide the full range of financing options, from fully insured to ASO. In thinking of the Blues, it is best to think of them as sixty-nine Blue Cross plans and sixty-nine Blue Shield plans, some considerably more efficient than others; in fiscal year 1976 the administrative cost per claim of Blue Shield plans involved in Medicare part B ranged from $1.90 for Rhode Island Blue Shield to $4.77 for Delaware Blue Shield.[18] In their private business some Blues plans charge nearly four times as much to process business claims as other plans charge (see box).[19] The Blues should be encouraged to compete against one another for business. Firms with employees in several geographic areas can fruitfully solicit bids from the Blues plans in all these areas. This is more easily achieved by working with the individual plans directly rather than through their national association.

The entry of data processing firms into health benefit program administration has increased competition for government contracts. The results of this competition are startling. Administrative cost savings of 20 percent and more have been achieved in the Medicaid and CHAMPUS contracts. One can speculate that such savings played a role in motivating HEW Secretary Joseph Califano to announce on April 12, 1978, the introduction of competitive bidding for Medicare part A contracts and to sharply increase competition under part B.[20]

In short, competitive bidding can save money. Serious consideration should be given to preparing a request for proposals (RFP) and soliciting as many qualified bidders as possible when an insurance or administrative contract is up for renewal. The review expense will be repaid both in dollar savings and in learning experience. In a recent RFP issued by the UMWA Health and Retirement Funds for the administration (ASO structure) of its new vision care program, the range in proposed costs among the three bidders judged most capable of providing the specified level of services was over 300 percent. Considerable preparation time and expense can be saved by modifying the model RFPs that are readily available from a number of sources, including the HEW Health Care Financing Administration, Medicaid state agencies, vendors, and the authors. In evaluating responses to RFPs, one area to study closely is the method for paying the contractor. Payments can be made in several ways including fixed amount, fixed amount per claim, variable amount dependent upon claim volumes, percentages of claims expenditures, and unit charge per covered employee and dependent. Special cognizance of the incentives created by the method of payment is highly advisable.

For example, the most common payment method for ASO contracts is based on percentage of claim expenditures. This means the more a contractor spends on claims, the more he earns; and he loses income whenever a claim is denied. The incentives ought instead to be aligned so that the contractor earns more by saving the clients more. Performance goals related to speed, accuracy, and thoroughness of processing in the contract are an excellent means of establishing incentives for effective administration.

As important as claims processing capabilities in selecting an administrative option is the level and quality of beneficiary services. Do beneficiaries get prompt, understandable, and relevant responses to written, telephone, and walk-in inquiries? Is the payment mechanism chosen by the carrier predominantly one that puts the burden on the beneficiary for record keeping and submission of bills or does it accept assignment by hospitals and physicians so that the beneficiaries' participation in the administrative process is minimal or absent. If the plan covers retirees who are likely to be Medicare eligible, has the system chosen an interface with the Medicare reimbursement process (particularly the part B carrier) which minimizes beneficiary inconvenience? Does the beneficiary receive assistance if needed in filling out claims forms? Is the

LOCAL BLUE CROSS-BLUE SHIELD PLAN SUBSCRIPTION REVENUES AND CLAIMS PAID
First Nine Months of 1977, in thousands of dollars

Plan	Subscription Revenue	Claims Paid	(Subscription Revenue ± Claims Paid) × 100
Worthington (BS only)	$225,421	$166,800	74.0
Denver (BS only)	42,605	33,373	78.3
Ranoke (BS only)	15,768	12,805	81.2
Cleveland (BS only)	93,598	76,640	81.9
Camp Hill (BS only)	360,047	300,764	83.5
Denver (BC only)	101,165	86,498	85.5
Allentown (BC only)	42,862	36,692	85.6
Louisville (Jt.)	195,658	169,273	86.5
Charleston (BS only)	10,764	9,340	86.8
Rockford (BC only)	36,021	31,590	87.7
Morgantown (BS only)	280	247	88.2
Salt Lake City (BS only)	26,098	23,040	88.3
Wheeling (BS only)	7,045	6,283	89.2
Cleveland (BS only)	254,218	229,447	90.3
Roanoke (BC only)	37,669	34,040	90.4
Richmond (BC only)	153,030	139,474	91.1
Richmond (BS only)	81,295	74,401	91.5
Philadelphia (BC only)	293,982	270,457	92.0
Columbus (BC only)	82,035	75,918	92.5
Pittsburg (BC only)	327,012	302,831	92.6
Salt Lake City (BC only)	35,394	32,815	92.7
Wilkes-Barre (BC only)	66,110	61,319	92.8
Toledo (BC only)	101,272	95,050	93.9
Indianapolis (BS only)	124,538	116,917	93.9
Clarksburg (BS only)	864	812	94.0
Parkersburg (BS only)	1,941	1,830	94.3
Chicago (Jt.)	603,990	573,330	94.9
Charleston (BC only)	29,677	28,207	95.0
Cincinnati (BC only)	307,641	292,774	95.2
Parkersburg (BC only)	6,097	5,882	96.5
Birmingham (Jt.)	209,311	202,417	96.7
Indianapolis (BC only)	242,882	235,228	96.9
Harrisburg (BC only)	98,949	96,343	97.4
Wheeling (BC only)	24,180	27,476	113.6

SOURCE: Provided by Blue Cross Association to United Mine Workers of America Health and Retirement Funds, January 1977.

carrier's description of benefits clear and understandable? Are useful and timely explanations of benefits provided?

Generally, and perhaps unfortunately, excluded from services is the concept of assisting the beneficiary in choosing a provider and helping in the coordination of care—the advocacy function. Somewhat more common are indirect efforts at beneficiary services, for instance, brochures and advertisements that speak of how to use the delivery system or how to stay healthy. These indirect interventions are too often simplistic and remote from people facing day-to-day illness who need help

Thus far we have discussed savings that may accrue to industry from control of administrative costs. However, because these costs rarely exceed 10 percent of total health expenditures, the savings potential here is limited. Far larger savings may be realized by adopting some of the approaches outlined in the next three sections in relation to structuring and managing the benefit package, and intervening in the health delivery system.

Structuring the Benefit Package

Employee education is vital. As changes in the structure of the benefit package are made, employees must understand them and accept their rationale. Specifically, employees must fully appreciate that excess costs come not only out of the employer's pocket but also out of their own and that this is true whether health care is tax-financed, employer-financed, or employee-financed. This appreciation, coupled with the assurance that a fair share of savings will be returned to the employee, becomes absolutely essential as the benefit package is actively managed. Because efforts to intervene in the system usually constrain employee choices among providers, employee understanding and cooperation is crucial.

Intervention efforts in the form of structuring the benefit package can be guided by the following seven principles:

1. Remove all or substantially all financial risk to employees for catastrophic expenses.

2. Place physicians at financial risk for inappropriate hospitalization and unnecessary ambulatory care by providing incentives to employees for enrollment in HMOs.

3. Where enrollment in an HMO is not chosen or not possible, consider coinsurance for physician services as well as copayments and deductibles for selected hospital services.

4. In defining benefits and structuring incentives, make certain that ambulatory care coverage is sufficiently broad and hospital coverage sufficiently restrictive to minimize hospitalization for conditions that can be diagnosed and treated on an ambulatory basis.

5. Encourage, where appropriate, the use of nonphysician providers (nurse practitioners and physician assistants) in home, office, and institu-

tional settings. Reimburse for their services at a lower rate than physician services.

6. Provide the means, encouragement, and incentives for employees and their families to stay healthy. The usual health benefits program represents little more than casualty insurance: the employee is reimbursed for medical expenses incurred. The more often he is ill, the more the benefit is worth to him. In the minds of many, the less they utilize, the less the benefit is worth to them. Obviously, attitudes of this kind need to be changed if unnecessary coverage (e.g., spouse has insurance) and utilization is to be reduced. Do your employees fully understand what their "free" health insurance actually costs? Do you issue an explanation of benefits (EOB), that includes the cost of services provided, either with each claim or on a periodic summary basis? Have you suggested to employees that savings achieved in this area could conceivably be shared through increased wages or other benefits? In summary, do your employees have a stake in staying healthy and utilizing medical benefits appropriately?

The benefit package should also include age- and service-specific preventive measures that have demonstrated their cost effectiveness. Screening should be limited to easily identified conditions where treatment has a good chance of favorably affecting outcome. The Breslow-Somers "Lifetime Health-Monitoring Program"[21] is an excellent starting point for discussing necessary inclusions.

7. Dental, vision, mental health, and drug benefits generally need rigorous management to prevent provider and patient abuse. These benefits will not be further discussed in this chapter except to note that the same principles of benefit package structuring, management, and systems intervention apply. For the most cost-effective delivery (that is, with costs contained and quality reasonable), vigorous and informed intervention is a prerequisite for success.

Managing the Benefit Package

Benefit management identifies areas of high use and determines whether these services were actually needed. Employees should react positively to such a program if it is properly explained and the point conveyed that unnecessary exposure to the medical system, particularly hospitals and surgery, is dangerous to employee health and employer's purse.

Benefit management requires analysts with professional training in health care to identify data areas of special concern. The next step is to inquire directly of providers, sometimes making visits to hospitals and physicians, to find the reason for a particular pattern of utilization or the justification of a pattern of practice—even to the point of assessing individual cases and their management. The assessment of individual cases should, wherever possible, have a prospective orientation. Retrospective denials of payment or inquiries that carry with them a perceived threat of malpractice litigation generate substantial anxiety and hostility in providers. It is well to keep in mind that the money to be saved by changing a pattern of behavior prospectively is almost always far greater than the money that would be recouped from renegotiating an expense already incurred. Analysis should not be designed to pinpoint past fault or error. Rather, the employer or carrier should view the discussion with the specific physician or hospital as directed toward gaining a better understanding of a pattern of practice. Of course, cases will arise where the behavior of a given hospital or physician is so outrageous that a carrier or an employer has a moral responsibility that goes beyond protecting its own policyholder or beneficiaries. In those, one hopes rare, cases, appropriate state and federal licensure and regulatory authorities must be notified.

Practice patterns may be categorized as (1) acceptable without change; (2) easily made mutually acceptable; or (3) outside the bounds of what a particular employer or carrier wishes to purchase. When a practice pattern falls into category (2) or (3), intervention can be either direct (to and through the patient or through providers) or indirect (through local professional standards review organizations (PSROs), medical societies, state licensing bodies, or national accreditation organizations). This discussion focuses particularly on direct interventions with physicians and hospitals, as it is here the purchasing power of industry is directly felt. Furthermore, it is the administrative and professional choice of providers that largely determines health care costs in any particular situation.

To be comprehensive, benefit management should have both reactive and anticipatory components. Both will affect either cost or quality and in most cases both.

Reactive management entails taking action based on analysis of past provider and patient behavior. For instance, Dr. Jones is performing more hysterectomies than his colleagues. Therefore let's take a look. Or Mr. Smith has seen a large number of physicians in a short period of time and is purchasing a large number of mood-altering drugs. Therefore, one might consider informing the physicians of Mr. Smith's behavior, however, invasion of privacy and confidentiality are clear concerns here.

Anticipatory management entails taking action before services are delivered. A firm might decide, for example:

That the value of peripheral vasodilators is so marginal or even negative that these drugs will not be covered in the benefits plan.

That open heart surgery performed in units handling fewer than 250 cases per year pose an unnecessary threat to the survival of patients, and that such a procedure in any such unit will not be covered.

That generic drugs are fully equivalent to and generally less expensive than their brand name counterparts, and the plan will reimburse only for drugs on fee schedules based on generic prices.

That because the ownership of hospital, nursing home, laboratory, and drug company stocks by physicians can influence their decisions about patient care, all physicians who do more than a certain dollar volume of business should be required to disclose all medically related investments that might affect patient care decisions. Those choosing not to disclose will not be eligible for reimbursement. Those whose disclosures reveal an apparent conflict will be subject to close scrutiny through ongoing surveillance and utilization review.

That hospital charges will be determined and agreed to before the fact for units of service that are difficult to distort. Inclusive fixed hospital per diems can then be negotiated to include all room, board and ancillary charges, rather than simply accepting fees for such charges with no control over the total cost per day in the hospital.

These kinds of interventions have three principal effects:

1.   The sentinel effect: people are more likely to think before acting if they know someone else is making a judgment about their behavior. This is akin to a forced internal second opinion.

2.   Specific impact: provider Jones or patient Smith is directly touched, and in some percentage of the cases a change in behavior will take place.

3.   Systems impact: with the passage of time and in the aggregate, the first two effects result in changed performance characteristics of the overall delivery system.

Cost analysis, particularly hospital cost analysis, today too often focuses on small pieces of the pie rather than on the whole. For instance, room charges, laboratory fees, operating room and x-ray fees may all be scrutinized and even be "low." However, if length of stay is up or ancillaries are numerous, then "low" becomes meaningless. Specifically, for employees of the same age group and sex, what is the total cost of hospitalization in hospital A versus hospital B versus hospital C for a particular rather standard procedure or illness such as gall bladder removal, hysterectomy, hernia repair, or acute myocardial infarction? Table 9 in the appendix shows that the cost variation among hospitals may be considerable. If, after considering such factors as access to care, availiabity of comparable services, physician admitting privileges, and age and sex structure of the patient population, there is no good explanation of the cost variation, then why not move toward limiting purchases from hospitals to those with lower total cost per case?

In high density areas specific provider agreements with selected hospitals and physicians may be appropriate. In the case of hospitals these agreements must either set or move toward a comprehensive definition of all costs associated with a day of care as well as speaking to admissions control and length of stay control. Physician agreements should be based on need for the services, qualifications, cost of service, clear willingness to maximize ambulatory care, and agreement to a limited number of critical restrictions—for instance, selected prior approvals, willingness to use prescription forms that instruct the pharmacist to dispense generic products where available unless the prescribing physician specifically indicates to the contrary, and administrative compliance such as charging and collecting coinsurance rather than forgiving such charges and raising fees. Financial rewards should be made to physicians who comply with performance goals, particularly in the area of controlling hospital admissions.

As a firm begins to select among providers, it is important to start slowly and have criteria in hand that are understood and supported not only within the firm but by some respected and credible members of the medical and hospital communities. Selection should be on the basis of patterns of practice and cost, placing equal emphasis on quality and cost concerns. Employees should always be left a very real choice of approved providers and a clear explanation of why a particular provider is not available. Concurrently, employees should be given direction and guidance to approved providers. Further, the employer or carrier should always make it perfectly clear that beneficiaries may go wherever they wish even though the carrier or company will not help them pay bills from an unacceptable provider. This type of approach, coupled with positive incentives to join HMOs, is practical, fair to all parties, and can work.

Intervening in the Health Delivery System

Interventions into the delivery system have as their primary objective changing the overall pattern of behavior of providers and patients. They are designed to affect all providers or large classes of providers and, in like manner, all patients or large classes of patients. This is different from interventions focused on a single provider which, if enough of them are made, can in the aggregate have a noticeable effect on the larger system. For instance, reducing hospital beds to control high utilization is a systems intervention. Identifying and interacting with individual physicians whose practices involve high admission rates and/or long lengths of stay is an individual intervention which will have a system effect only if it causes large numbers of providers to significantly change their behavior.

Systems interventions have thus far, for all practical purposes, been left to the government; rate setting, certificate of need, PSROs, and health planning (health systems agencies, state health coordinating councils, and state health planning and development agencies) are on the government regulatory and planning smorgasbord today. Carrier passivity in the realm of systems intervention has been and remains so marked that many feel that excessive medical care costs can be laid at the feet of carriers who essentially pay on demand. Without question, some carriers can give examples of worthwhile systems interventions. But too often, these have been fragmented and limited efforts which appear to be designed as much for public relations impact as for any substantive effect on cost and quality of care.

However, carrier passivity is understandable. Insurers want (and indeed, need) to satisfy clients, and unless clients—employers—require intervention, intervene they will not. Why? It's different, uncomfortable, and might even hurt carrier profits or the Blues' equivalent of profit. Further, carriers are not always neutral. The Blue Cross plans were in the past closely tied to hospitals and the Blue Shield plans are still close to if not controlled by physicians. Some private carriers have as major investments hospital capital development projects and may not vigorously pursue policies of admissions control or hospital cost control because this might adversely affect the financial viability of their investments. The life insurance side of a large multiple line carrier may be reluctant to have the health insurance side offend physicians, who tend to be in high income brackets and to buy substantial amounts of life insurance. Special purpose insurance companies covering drugs, vision, and dental care may either be owned by or be clear spinoffs of that segment of the industry they are designed to finance. Thus it is vital to know the history, background of directors, investment patterns, organizational philosophy, and the real source of ultimate organizational decisionmaking for each carrier a company may be considering. The answers to these questions must be weighed in the light of what a company expects of a particular carrier. If such questions are not addressed in a straightforward manner, there is real danger that unanticipated conflict of carrier interest will impede company efforts at cost control. The dangers are obvious.

Systems interventions are thoughtfully discussed in the first volume of the Springer Series on Industry and Health Care.[22] They are of two basic types: supportive or active. Supportive activities are those where an industry or carrier participates in and lends support to someone else's efforts, for instance, participating in a health systems agency or joining the board of a local HMO. Active involvement implies doing something that has a measurable result, where success or failure can be more readily if not easily discerned by management, the public, and providers. Examples are: making a corporate commitment of staff and money to the development of selected HMOs; requiring the carrier to develop plans and implementation strategy including specific milestones and measurable objectives with the goal of reducing hospitalization by x percent in y years (x must be greater than any natural rate of decline); or developing and using specific quantitative criteria for the performance of the delivery system as it affects your employee populations.

For example, you may conclude that males in the 15–44 age group require for good care only x days per person per year of inpatient medical and surgical services. In addition, you have made similar conclusions for men and women under age 15, women age 15–44, men and women in the 45–65 age group, as well as the over-65 group. Taken together, these policy standards allow you to determine the number of bed days of hospital care you should be buying for your employees. When considered in conjunction with the total population of a community, it allows for forecasting of bed needs.[23] In an analogous manner, physician need in the aggregate and by specialty can be calculated. These conclusions can be used by the firm or the carrier to manage the benefit package to move your employee utilization to conform to the established policy goals, or to support and intervene in the planning, regulatory, and rate-setting processes to bring about patterns of capital development, reimbursement, and physician migration to meet the goals.

Both mean, among other things, choosing among providers, particularly hospitals, It is not sufficient to reduce utilization and end up with empty but open beds. That's costly. Rather, as hospital utilization declines, the remaining use must be targeted at fewer hospitals so that they may function in a cost-effective manner. If utilization goes down and bed capacity remains static, hospitals will stay open, overstaffed, and underutilized, and will still contribute substantially to needless cost. This may enhance quality, because unnecessary hospitalization has been prevented. However, it achieves almost nothing with regard to control of cost.[24]

Any system for intervention should recognize the practical reality that doctors practicing alone and in small groups will be the predominant system of care for years to come. HMOs of two types, individual practice associations (IPAs) and prepaid group practice plans (PPGPs), will continue to grow. However, the IPA,[25] which uses as its base the do tor already in practice with his existing office and often many of his current patients, probably has the greater chance for growth than PPGPs of the Kaiser type. Why? Simply because the IPA requires less change on the part of the physician and the patient.

Physicians may choose various types of organizations in which to practice, for example, individual and small group practices, health centers, nurse practitioner satellite clinics, hospital-based ambulatory care programs, or the various types of HMOs. Whatever the practice format, it is appropriate to discriminate between those who are both acceptable and needed and those that are either unacceptable or unneeded. The former meet initial tests of reasonable cost and need as well as ongoing compliance with cost, consumer satisfaction, and administrative criteria. On the other hand, physicians may be unacceptable or unneeded because they have excessively costly or grossly aberrant patterns of practice, because they are administratively noncompliant, or generate extensive consumer dissatisfaction or are clearly in oversupply.

Hospitals can be dichotomized in a similar manner on the basis of costs, need, patient acceptance, patterns of service, utilization, and administrative compliance. Discriminating among providers in these ways stimulates provider performance and competition while broadening the real options available to purchaser and patient.

The range and mix of interventions a particular company may choose from the five broad categories of cash flow management, choice of administrative mechanisms, structuring the benefit package, managing the benefit package, and intervening in the health delivery system will appropriately vary according to the unique circumstances that surround it. A firm may choose a strategy ranging from minimal through modest to very active. Different companies and the same company at different stages in the development of a health care cost containment strategy will choose different interventions.

Organizing to Intervene

How can individual companies and, more generally, industry organize to intervene effectively and what specific steps should be considered? A company wants to intervene to both manage benefits and affect the larger delivery system. What can be done to implement such a decision?

A necessary precondition is acceptance by top corporate management of the need to intervene in the personal health services delivery system in order to contain costs. This acceptance should carry with it a full understanding that payoff in terms of real cost control will take time. An initial commitment of several years' resources that is linked to specific realistic objectives and milestones is a helpful management device. This will foster rational staffing decisions and establish a framework for periodic evaluations. As the task will be difficult, particularly in the first few years, reassessment and, where appropriate, modification of objectives and milestones should be an integral part of ongoing program evaluation.

A critical component of any decision to intervene is to understand the need for data and to take steps to obtain a minimum data set. Only through having basic cost, utilization, and population data that can be compared over time with others' experience and one's own can informed management decisions be made.

Illustrative options for organizing include:

1.   The minimum model: existing or only slightly enhanced staff capacity with moderate to heavy use of outside consultants.

2.   The in-house model: enhanced corporate staff capacity. Whether one monitors carrier performance or opts for self-administration, enhanced staff capacity is likely to be needed.

3.   The carrier requirements model: the company develops performance requirements and reporting procedures for benefits management and systems intervention by its carrier(s). These requirements and procedures go well beyond the mere specification of accuracy and timeliness for claims processing and speak to utilization and cost targets as well as health planning interventions to be achieved by specific dates. Incentive reimbursements to carriers, providers, and employees could be linked to successful achievement of specific objectives.

4.   The consortium model: multicompany, multi-industry health consortia formed in areas of common medical interest. In this case organizations in a given medical trade area who may otherwise have no common interest—for instance, a home appliance manufacturer, a union trust fund, and a construction equipment company—would join together for purposes of improving the cost effectiveness of service delivery. How might such new groups organize? First, they would identify geographic areas where such approaches are possible. Thus the company or group initially interested in intervention has as a part of its work program the identification of other large employers or representatives of employee groups in the relevant medical trade area. The second step—logical but not necessarily easy—is to interest and involve the other large organizations. Involvement could be on an ad hoc basis, through a formal local consortium arrangement, or could even develop to the point where an appropriate legal vehicle was created through which technical assistance and planning funds could be channeled. Ultimately, such a group might become the agent for purchasing services and be viewed by the provider community as a broker that had to be listened to and satisfied if purchase

dollars from individual organizations were to come their way in the quantities desired.

The carrier requirements model could well involve but would not be limited to working with planning agencies, particularly health systems agencies. The consortium model can complement and strengthen planning agencies, but in concept it goes beyond the consensual and all to often provider-oriented decision making of these bodies. PSROs, by virtue of their control by local physicians, are no substitute for company initiative and responsibility.

Enhancement of staff capacity and modification of organizational structure within a particular company may often be a necessary antecedent to any effort at intervention. For maximum impact it will, in some cases, be necessary and appropriate to look outside a particular company and identify other large purchasers of service whose technical skills, political influence, and purchasing power in a given area, when combined with your company's strength, are such that planning agencies and the provider community will not only listen but respond.

What are the skills that a corporation must have available to it, either staff or consultative, if it wants to intervene? Certainly, legal (emphasis areas include antitrust and tax as well as federal and state health regulatory and planning law), actuarial, health care finance, health systems development and planning talent is needed, as is the capacity to interpret medical judgments and take positions on changing technologies and procedures.

To what extent need physicians be involved in employers' interventions in the health system? Carefully selected and appropriately trained nonphysicians can do much of the job. For instance, nurse practitioners, public health graduates with work experience in clinical settings, hospital administrators, and social workers are all good lower cost candidates. Physician backup is required, both for intermittent consultation and supervision of corporate staff as well as for occasional frontline presence where a doctor-to-doctor encounter is necessary. Special training for physicians in data analysis as well as intervention skills may be necessary.

An additional value of physician availability in the intervention process is the nonphysician staff are stronger and surer when they know that if a showdown comes they can call on and get a physician's support. This support goes beyond technical assistance in particular substance areas. It is also useful in physician-nonphysician communications. In a confrontation with physicians, nonphysicians may encounter such postures as: "Do you want to take the responsibility for my patients? . . . for practicing medicine? . . . for deaths this approach will cost?" Such tactics are tempting for the physician to use and difficult for the nonphysician to resist, whatever the merits of the case. Use of another physician in such discussions helps disarm unwarranted tactics.

However organized, the corporate staff must work as a team with common goals, together thrashing out approaches that have the best chance of working. Catalyzing and coordinating such a team effort between widely disparate disciplines is crucial if intervention is to be meaningful and cost containment effective.

Summary

The highlights of successful cost containment of the health benefit include:

Corporate management must both understand and support intervention.

Modest in-house capacity, with or without consultative assistance, must include legal, financial analysis, health system, and medical skills.

Data—who gets what services, where, provided by whom, and at what cost—are essential.

Standard reporting requirements for in-house health benefit managers or carriers ought to be developed.

Business skills and knowledge can be employed to manage cash and encourage competition among carriers and providers.

Where appropriate a switch should be made from fully insured to the less costly financing structures.

Self-insurance and self-administration should be considered.

Savings from interventions must be shared with employees.

Benefit package performance requirements should be established that address utilization and costs.

Multicompany consortia might be organized in geographic areas of common medical interest.

Intervention to any degree can save money and improve services. Each admission prevented saves $500 to $1,000 or more. Reducing hospitalization by only 0.1 day per beneficiary per year saves at least $200,000 for every 10,000 beneficiaries. The bigger the investment, the greater the likely return. Difficult? Yes. Different? Yes. Needed for companies, employees, and the country? Without question, yes.

NOTES

1. Office of Management and Budget, *Special Analysis, Budget of the U.S. Government, 1979*, Washington, D.C., January 1978, p. 242.

2. Ibid.

3. Calculated from Health Insurance Institute news release, February 16, 1978; $623/day in 1976 adjusted for 16 percent increase for 1977 per *Medicare-Medicaid Information*, vol. 3, no. 3 (March 1978), p. 9.

4. Department of Health, Education and Welfare, *Health: United States*, 1976–1977, table 169.

5. *Medicare-Medicaid Information* (March 1978), p. 8.

6. Between 1950 and 1976 total health expenditures increased at an average annual rate of 919 percent, but at only 4.9 percent adjusted for inflation.

7. Office of Management and Budget, *Special Analysis*, p. 242.

8. Ibid.

9. Victor R. Fuchs, *Who Shall Live* (New York: Basic Books, 1974).

10. *Mercer Bulletin*, vol. 4, no. 4 (April 1978).

11. Ibid. Calculation based on 33 percent direct pays in 1976.

12. *Federal Register*, September 17, 1976, p. 40319.

13. *Health: United States, 1976–1977*, p. 348.

14. Ibid.

15. "Approval Program for Blue Cross Plans," courtesy of Blue Cross Association.

16. Blue Cross Association Management Summary Report to Chief Plan Executives, 1976.

17. Executive Office of the President, Council on Wage and Price Stability, *The Complex Puzzle of Rising Health Care Costs: Can the Private Sector Fit it Together?* (Washington, D.C.: USGPO, December 1976), p. iv.

18. From Department of Health, Education and Welfare, 1977 "Analysis of Intermediaries and Carriers Administrative Costs," Washington, D.C.

19. "Comparison of Unit Costs and National Performance Standards Data, Third Quarter 1977," Blue Cross Association, January 31, 1978.

20. Department of Health, Education and Welfare press release, April 12, 1978.

21. *New England Journal of Medicine*, vol. 296 (1977), pp. 601–608.

22. D.C. Walsh and R.H. Egdahl, *Payer, Provider, Consumer: Industry Confronts Health Care Costs* (New York: Springer-Verlag, 1977).

23. D.C. Walsh and W.J. Bicknell, "Forecasting the Need for Hospital Beds: A Quantitative Methodology," *Public Health Reports*, vol. 92 (1977), pp. 199–210.

24. W. McClure, "Reducing Excess Hospital Capacity," DHEW (HRA-230-0086), October 15, 1976.

25. R.H. Egdahl et al., "The Potential of Organizations of Fee-for-Service Physicians for Achieving Significant Decreases in Hospitalization," *Annals of Surgery*, vol. 186 (1977), pp. 156–167.

Appendix: An Illustrative Data Base for System Intervention

Tables 1 through 9 provide data from national sources and from the United Mine Workers of America Health and Retirement Funds, to illustrate the data elements needed in order to plan effective intervention into the delivery system: expenditure data (table 1), population data, by age, sex, and geographical location (tables 2 through 5), utilization data (table 6), resource data (tables 7 and 8), and cost data (table 9).

Table 1
Illustrative Expenditure Data (in millions of dollars)

Program (FY)	Hospital	Physician	Other	Total	Per Capita
United States (1976) [a]	55,400 (40%)	26,350 (19%)	57,562 (41%)	139,312	638
Medicare (1975) [b]	10,316 (72%)	3,269 (23%)	757 (5%)	14,342	831 for 1977
Medicaid (1976) [c]	4,518 (32%)	1,387 (10%)	8,340 (58%)	14,245	753 for 1977
Federal Employees Program (CY 1978) [d]	High Option Family Coverage				1,336
Canadian Health Service [e]					858
Public Health Service [e]					730
UMWA HRF (1975) [f]	(47%)	106 (48%)	19 (9%)	220	360 ($840 family)
Blue Cross–Blue Shield of N.C., [g] Premiums effective May 1, 1977				family	1,304
Health Maintenance Plan–Cincinnati (1977) [h]				family	1,145
Group Health Plan of Northeast Ohio (1977) [h]				family	937
Blue Cross–Blue Shield of Ohio HMO (1977) [h]				family	929
Kansas Community Health Foundation–Cleveland (1977) [h]				family	899
Medical Foundation of Bellaire (1977) [h]				family	859
Georgetown University Community Health Plan (effective Oct. 1, 1978) [i]				family	1,286

a. M. S. Mueller and R. M. Gibson, "National Health Expenditures, Fiscal Year 1975," Social Security Bulletin 39(2) (February 1976) (Preliminary Estimates).
b. Office of Management and Budget, Special Analysis, Budget of the U.S. Government, 1979, January 1978, p. 246.
c. Ibid., p. 247.
d. Mike Causey, "Health Premiums Rise Looms," Washington Post, October 18, 1977, p. C2.
e. Eileen Connor, "Health Expenditure Comparisons, December 2, 1977 Estimates," from DHEW Working Document–Discussion Paper on Government Delivery of Health Services, October 23, 1977, authored by Delivery of Services Team for NHI, p. 1.
f. Ibid., p. 2 in conjunction with UMWA Health and Retirement Funds Financial Reports.
g. Rates charged for health coverage of UMWA Health and Retirement Funds employees by Group Hospitalization, Inc., and Medical Service of D.C.
h. Provided by Bellarie Clinic in proposal to UMWA HRF, June 25, 1977.
i. Provided by Georgetown Community Health Plan in proposal to UMWA HRF, August 8, 1978.

Table 2
Illustrative Utilization Data: Rate per 1,000 Population of Discharges, Days of Care, and Average Length of Stay in Nonfederal Short-Stay General Hospitals, United States, 1973

Age	Discharges	Days of Care	Average Length of Stay
Under 15	70.6	321.0	4.5
15–44	154.4	878.9	5.7
45–64	182.7	1665.2	9.1
65 and over	342.5	4144.8	12.1
Sex			
Male	129.3	1067.2	8.3
Female	180.8	1344.5	7.4

SOURCE: *The Nation's Use of Health Resources,* United States Department of Health, Education, and Welfare, Health Resources Administration (DHEW Publication No. HLA 77-1240) table 19, p. 48.

Table 3
Illustrative Utilization Data: Office Visits to Physicians, by Age and Sex of Patient, United States, 1974 (Civilian Noninstitutional Population)

	All Ages	Under 15	15–24	24–44	45–64	65 and over
Male	2.5	2.6	1.7	2.2	3.3	4.3
Female	3.6	2.1	3.3	4.0	4.2	5.0

SOURCE: USDEHEW, *Health, United States, 1976–1977,* table 80, p. 257.

Table 4
Illustrative Population Data: Location and Distribution of UMWA Funds Health Cardholders by State and County

	(1) Counties with 100 or More Cardholders	(2) Cardholders in Counties with 100 or More Cardholders	(3)[a] % Total Cardholders in State	(4) Cardholders in All Counties in State	(5) % Total Cardholders by State
West Virginia	38	82,654	99.4	83,161	30.4
Pennsylvania	17	52,818	98.9	53,414	19.6
Kentucky	27	32,717	97.0	33,715	12.4
Virginia	10	19,187	93.1	20,603	8.0
Illinois	23	18,510	93.3	19,834	7.3
Ohio	22	16,332	90.5	18,038	6.7
Alabama	10	13,456	97.0	13,898	5.1
Indiana	10	5,688	85.6	6,643	2.4
Tennessee	6	2,088	71.5	2,917	1.1
	163	243,450		249,304	93

SOURCE: United Mine Workers of America Health and Retirement Funds, unpublished working document, January 1, 1976.

[a]Column 2 divided by Column 4.

Table 5
Illustrative Population Data: Location and Distribution of UMWA Funds Health Cardholders in 38 West Virginia Counties with 100 or More Cardholders

100–499 Cardholders		500–1999 Cardholders		2000 or more Cardholders		Totals	
						Number	Percentage
Clay	(496)	Marshall	(1,603)	Raleigh	(9,953)		
Brooke	(463)	Greenbriar	(1,541)	McDowell	(8,989)		
Wetzer	(456)	Ohio	(1,365)	Logan	(7,470)		
Upshur	(437)	Barbour	(940)	Fayette	(6,600)		
Mason	(395)	Preston	(910)	Wyoming	(5,435)		
Taylor	(325)	Lincoln	(898)	Kanawha	(5,340)		
Wayne	(297)	Webster	(703)	Marion	(5,267)		
Tucker	(290)	Randolph	(521)	Boone	(4,832)		
Cabell	(258)			Mercer	(4,390)		
Summers	(245)			Mingo	(3,795)		
Braxton	(196)			Monongalia	(3,022)		
Tyler	(192)			Nicholas	(2,255)		
Grant	(143)			Harrison	(2,151)		
Putnam	(134)						
Jackson	(121)						
Mineral	(118)						
Lewis	(108)						
4,674		8,481		69,499			
						82,654	30.3	(38 West Virginia Counties)
						83,161	30.5	(All West Virginia)
						272,785	100	(Total UMWA Cardholders)

Table 6
Illustrative Comparative Utilization Data: UMWA Funds Totals Versus Other Totals

Plan	Physician Visits per Member per Year	Hospital Discharge per 1,000 per Year	Hospital Days per 1,000 per Year	Average Length of Stay
United States Total	5.1	141	924.5	6.58
Blue Cross Total (under 65)			808	6.70
Prepaid HMO Totals (U.S.)	3.8		449	
Funds Total (under 65)	4.2	176.6	1029	5.85
Northeast Region HMO Total	4.4		532	
Pa. Prepaid Total	3.8		799	
Funds, Johnstown Area		158.9	1025	6.21
North Central Region HMO Prepaid Total	3.6		547	
Indiana Prepaid Total	3.0		264	
Funds, Evansville Area		194.2	1092	5.62
Southern Region HMO Total	4.1		476	
West Va. HMO Total	5.0		690	
Funds, Beckley Area		190.1	1020	5.22
Western Region HMO Total	3.7		409	
Colorado HMO Total	2.7		386	
Funds, Denver Area		146.4	734	5.18

SOURCES: *U.S. Totals:* DHEW *Health, U.S., 1976–1977;* UMWA Funds Totals: *1975 Annual Medical Statistics,* UMWA Health and Retirement Funds; *HMO Totals:* National HMO Census (unpublished) 1976 Blue Cross Association, National Association of Blue Shield Plans Interstudy and Division of HMO-DHEW.

Table 7
Illustrative Resource Data: Physicians and Hospital Beds by State, 1974

State	Active Nonfederal Physicians per 100,000 Population	Short-Stay Nonfederal Hospital Beds per 1,000 Civilian Population[a]
Alabama	93	4.78
Alaska	85	2.25
Arizona	151	3.88
Arkansas	92	4.50
California	194	4.06
Colorado	169	4.21
Connecticut	202	3.54
Delaware	139	3.54
District of Columbia	429	7.02

(Continued)

Table 7 (*Continued*)
Illustrative Resource Data: Physicians and Hospital Beds by State, 1974

State	Active Nonfederal Physicians per 100,000 Population	Short-Stay Nonfederal Hospital Beds per 1,000 Civilian Population[a]
Florida	146	4.57
Georgia	106	4.31
Hawaii	155	3.22
Idaho	92	3.99
Illinois	151	4.90
Indiana	105	4.40
Iowa	103	5.96
Kansas	123	5.70
Kentucky	110	4.33
Louisiana	122	4.54
Maine	115	4.62
Maryland	199	3.22
Massachusetts	216	4.70
Michigan	132	4.43
Minnesota	157	5.98
Mississippi	86	4.76
Missouri	134	5.40
Montana	104	5.35
Nebraska	119	6.15
Nevada	112	4.39
New Hampshire	140	4.19
New Jersey	156	3.99
New Mexico	114	3.41
New York	236	4.77
North Carolina	116	4.08
North Dakota	94	6.87
Ohio	136	4.51
Oklahoma	101	4.57
Oregon	153	3.99
Pennsylvania	155	4.75
Rhode Island	172	3.77
South Carolina	101	3.99
South Dakota	78	5.61
Tennessee	127	5.16
Texas	121	4.66
Utah	145	3.20
Vermont	179	4.77
Virginia	131	4.00
Washington	152	3.49
West Virginia	111	5.78
Wisconsin	125	5.22
Wyoming	97	4.72
United States Total	152	4.54

SOURCES: DHEW, *Health U.S., 1976–1977, table 118, p. 314; table 127, p. 328.*
[a]Excluding psychiatric beds.

Table 8
Area Resource File Basic Area Profile

COUNTY: RALEIGH   WEST VIRGINIA

NUMBER OF COUNTIES	1
NUMBER SMSA COUNTIES	0
TOTAL LAND AREA	605

1974 POPULATION (000s)	75.5
1970 NO. HOUSEHOLDS (000s)	18.2
1970 % RURAL POPULATION	71.6
1974 POPULATION/SQ. MILE	125
1970 POP AS % OF 1960 POP	90.0

1970 PERCENTAGE BY RACE:

% WHITE	88.1
% BLACK	11.5
% INDIAN	0.1
% OTHER	0.3

1970 SEX-AGE DISTRIBUTION:

	TOTAL	0–4	5–14	15–24	25–34	35–44	45–54	55–64	65 & OVER
Total	100.0	8.0	19.2	16.9	9.8	11.0	12.6	10.9	11.5
% MALE	47.9	3.9	9.9	8.5	4.6	4.9	5.9	5.2	5.2
% FEMALE	52.1	4.2	9.3	8.5	5.2	6.2	6.7	5.7	6.3

POPULATION BY COUNTY TYPE AND SIZE:

	TOTAL	SMSA COUNTIES—BY SMSA SIZE		NON-SMSA COUNTIES—BY SIZE OF LARGEST CITY IN COUNTY		
		1 + MIL.	UNDER 1 MIL.	OVER 24999	5000–24999	UNDER 5000
NO. COUNTIES	1	0	0	0	1	0
% POPULATION	100.0	0.0	0.0	0.0	100.0	0.0

1970 PERSONAL INCOME ($ MIL.)	149.0
1970 PERSONAL INCOME/CAPITA	2125
1970 PERSONAL INCOME/HOUSEHOLD	8184
1970 INCOME/CAPITA AS % of 1960	187.0

1975 AID DEPENDENT CHILDREN POPULATION	2614
ADC POP./100000 TOTAL POPULATION	3462.3

1970 FAMILIES + UNRELATED INDIVIDUALS INCOME LEVELS:

	TOTAL	UNDER $3000	$3000–4999	$5000–9999	$10000 & OVER
% OF FAMILIES + UNRELATED INDIVIDUALS	100.0	30.5	17.0	32.7	19.8

	MEDICAL SCHOOLS	OSTEOPATHY SCHOOLS	DENTAL SCHOOLS	NURSING (RN) SCHOOLS	NURSING (LPN) SCHOOLS	DENTAL AUXILIARY SCHOOLS
NUMBER	0	0	0	0	1	0
ENROLLMENT	0	0	0	0	36	0
GRADUATES	0	0	0	0	30	0

NUMBER MEDICAL SCHOOLS
(CONTINUING EDUCATION COURSES) 0   PER 100 MDS .... 0)

NUMBER MEDICAL AUXILIARY SCHOOLS 2   CAPACITY OF PROGRAM 16

NUMBER OPTOMETRY SCHOOLS 0
NUMBER PHARMACY SCHOOLS 0
NUMBER PODIATRY SCHOOLS 0
NUMBER VETERINARY SCHOOLS 0

NUMBER UNIVERSITIES ... 0   NUMBER COLLEGES 1   NUMBER JR. COLLEGES 1

	TOTAL	PER 100000 POPULATION	PER $100000 INCOME
1973 ACTIVE PHYSICIANS (MD) ...	112	149	0.075
1971 ACTIVE PHYSICIANS (OD) ...	6	9	0.004
TOTAL PHYSICIANS	118	158	0.079
1974 LICENSED DENTISTS	24	31	0.016

1972 OPTOMETRISTS 4
1973/74 PHARMACISTS 26
1974 PODIATRISTS 1

PER 100 HOSPITALS BEDS (GEN. & SPEC.)   1975 VETERINARIANS 4

1972 NURSES (RN)	239	341	32.7
1967 NURSES (LPN)	294	419	40.2
TOTAL NURSES	533	760	72.8

1974 NUMBER GENERAL HOSPITALS 4
(NUMBER BEDS/HOSPITAL .... 183)
(NUMBER BEDS/100000 PCP .... 970)

DISTRIBUTION OF GENERAL HOSPITALS:

BY NO. BEDS:	TOTAL	0–99	100–99	200–99	300–99	400+
	4	0	2	2	0	0

% UTILIZATION:	0–69%	70–79%	80–89%	90% +
	2	0	0	2

NUMBER OTHER HOSPITALS 0

AMA ACCREDITED TRAINING

NUMBER OF INTERN PROGRAMS 0   NUMBER OF INTERNSHIPS OFFERED . 0
NUMBER OF RESIDENCY PROGRAMS .. 1   NUMBER OF RESIDENCIES OFFERED .. 15

(Continued)

Table 8 (Continued)
Area Resource File Basic Area Profile

ALL HOSPITALS

NUMBER IN FAMILY MEDICINE	0	NUMBER OFFERED	0
NUMBER IN INTERNAL MEDICINE	0	NUMBER OFFERED	0
NUMBER IN PEDIATRIC	1	NUMBER OFFERED	3
NUMBER IN OBS. & GYN	0	NUMBER OFFERED	0

1974 NUMBER OF GENERAL HOSPITALS WITH GIVEN SERVICES:

INTENSIVE CARE	3	ELECTROENCEPHALOGRAPHY	2	PSYCHIATRIC-PART. HOSP	1
INTENSIVE CARDIAC	3	PHYSICAL THERAPY	4	PSYCHIATRIC-EMERGENCY	1
OPEN HEART SURGERY	0	OCCUPATIONAL THERAPY	0	SOCIAL WORK	1
RECOVERY ROOM	4	INHALATION THERAPY	4	FAMILY PLANNING	3
PREMATURE NURSERY	2	F-T REG. PHARMACIST	4	EXTENDED CAFE	0
X-RAY THERAPY	1	P-T REG. PHARMACIST	0	REHABILITATION-INPATIENT	1
COBALT THERAPY	0	DIALYSIS-INPATIENT	0	REHABILITATION-OUTPATIENT	0
RADIUM THERAPY	0	DIALYSIS-OUTPATIENT	1	HOME CARE	1
RADIOISTOPE THERAPY	2	SELF-CARE UNIT	0	HOSPITAL AUXILIARY	0
HISTOPATHOLOGY LABORATORY	4	PSYCHIATRIC FOSTER CARE	0	ORGANIZED OUTPATIENT DEPT.	1
ORGAN BANK	0	PSYCHIATRIC-INPATIENT	0	ABORTION (INPATIENT)	0
BLOOD BANK	2	PSYCHIATRIC-OUTPATIENT	2	ABORTION (OUTPATIENT)	0

DISTRIBUTION OF GENERAL HOSPITALS BY SERVICES OFFERED:

NUMBER OF SERVICES:	0–4	5–14	15–24	25 +
	0	3	1	0

LEVEL OF EMERGENCY SERVICE: MAJOR DEPARTMENT 3 MINOR DEPARTMENT 0 BASIC UNIT 1 REFERRAL ONLY . 0

NUMBER OUTPATIENT VISITS	93470	NUMBER INPATIENT DAYS	201950
OUTPATIENT VISITS/100000 POP	123801	INPATIENT DAYS/100000 POP	267483
% CHANGE OUTPATIENT VISITS 1973–1974	26	% CHANGE INPATIENT DAYS 1973–1974	11

1969–73 5-YR INFANT MORTALITY RATE/1000 BIRTHS 21.8   1974 MORTALITY PER 100000 POP 1170.9

SOURCE: HEW, *The Area Resource File: A Manpower Planning and Research Tool*, 1976

Table 9
Illustrative Comparative Cost Data: Annual Discharges, Average Length of Stay, Average Cost per Hospital Case, and Average Cost per Day for Cholecystectomy in High-Volume Hospitals in a Common Medical Trade Area[a]

Hospitals	No. of Cases Discharges[b]	Average Length of Stay	Average Total Hospital Cost	Average Cost per Day
A	9	16.6	$2404	$145
B	12	10.8	1417	131
C	18	12.3	1998	162
D	18	10.4	1159	111
E	6	9.0	920	102
	63	11.7	$1610	$137

[a]Non-Medicare Patients Only.
[b]Discharges are similar to admissions but exclude deaths.
SOURCE: Actual Annualized Data From the Four 1977 Quarterly Runs of The UMWA Health and Retirement Funds' Automated Surveillance and Utilization Review System.

Legal Considerations

John D. Blum

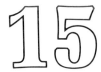

Corporations attempting to restructure employee health benefit plans may encounter certain legal problems, depending on the nature of the specific changes contemplated and on whether those changes are to be undertaken as sole or joint ventures. Because of the diversity of corporate approaches to employee health care, this chapter can only serve to outline some general areas of the law that need to be considered in restructuring health plans. Specifically, it addresses antitrust, preemption of state regulation under the Employee Retirement Income Security Act (ERISA), and confidentiality of medical records. These areas do not exhaust the legal questions companies could encounter in their efforts to reduce health care expenditures, but each is a major legal problem area and serves to highlight the complex ramifications under law that could result from misdirected use of corporate power in the health care system.

Antitrust

Antitrust is the body of law, both common and statutory, that is concerned with controlling private economic power by fostering competition. (See box.) The heart of antitrust enforcement lies in the application of three federal statutes: the Sherman Act,[1] which forbids contracts, combinations, or conspiracies in restraint of trade and prohibits interstate monopolies; the Clayton Act,[2] which restricts buyer-seller "tie-in" arrangements and prohibits anticompetitive mergers and acquisitions; and the Federal Trade Commission Act,[3] which prohibits unfair and deceptive methods of competition. The states have comparable legislation modeled after federal law to deal with intrastate antitrust problems. In evaluating the antitrust challenge raised by corporate health care cost reduction efforts either by one company or a group, one should give particular attention to the issues of restraint of trade and monopoly, both of which are violations of the Sherman Act.

Restraint of Trade

Restraint of trade includes a wide range of violations, whether they be contracts, combinations, or conspiracies, designed to reduce competition and obtain a dominant market position. Actions that constitute restraint of trade violations may be "per se" illegal if they have been so deemed by a court (such as price fixing among competitors).[4] In cases that do not fit into the "per se" violation category, courts apply the "rule of reason" to evaluate violations. This "rule" allows certain types of restraints to exist; situations are evaluated on a case-by-case basis with an eye toward the market power and the likely effects of a given combination. If a restraint is viewed as "undue," then it will be found violative of antitrust law.

In the health benefits context, restraints could arise from certain carrier-corporate agreements. If, however, there is an overriding valid commercial purpose in a particular arrangement—for example, reduction of health care premium costs—its restrictive aspects may be viewed as ancillary restraints even if they may normally constitute "per se" violations. Ancillary restraints are evaluated under the "rule of reason" and judged lawful if the restraint is reasonable, that is, necessary to the primary legitimate purpose of the arrangement, and does not unreasonably affect competition or is not imposed by a party with monopoly power.[5]

An example of a situation where evaluation of an ancillary restraint is pertinent is in fee schedule arrangements negotiated between corporations and insurers where one of the parties is supporting use of a fixed maximum fee schedule.[6] There is nothing "per se" illegal about third parties' use of fee schedules to evaluate the reasonableness of charges, but a restraint of trade challenge may be brought where an insurer is pressured by one or more corporate purchasers into developing a given fee schedule:[7] such use of dominant corporate power over the marketplace, if it seems to restrict price competition, is potentially violative of antitrust law. However, a given fee arrangement may be seen as only an ancillary restraint if its negative aspects are outweighed by its reasonableness and its ultimate ability to effectuate cost savings without seriously reducing competition.

In the restraint of trade area the violation most directly relevant to corporate health plans is price fixing. In situations where corporations or business consortiums have the ability to use their purchasing power to set fees, such action may be found illegal. While the judicial interpretations of what constitutes price fixing have been broad, it is clear that the activity must go beyond the power of a corporation to negotiate fee arrangements and reach a situation where the actor in question has actually dictated fee levels. An example of a price-fixing challenge can be seen in a recent court action in which the United Mine Workers Welfare and Retirement Fund* was accused by one of its participating hospitals of violating federal antitrust laws.[8] The fund had established a maximum per diem price for hospital services and specified that beneficiaries could not be required to pay the differences between the per diem rate and the hospital's standard charge. The plaintiff hospital attempted unilaterally to raise its charges, but the defendant union fund would only pay its pro rata share of what it considered to be justified increases. The fund informed the hospital that unless a mutually satisfactory price arrangement was agreed upon, hospitalization of fund beneficiaries would be restricted to emergencies only. The court found the restraint of trade challenge without merit. The fund's role in negotiating a price for medical care on behalf of beneficiaries was viewed by the court as similar to a group buying agent. The court did indicate that such a welfare fund is not precluded from antitrust law coverage; however, nothing present in this fund's particular conduct could be construed as a restraint of trade violation.

Monopsony

Monopoly is the use of market power to control prices or exclude competition.[9] It is most often a situation in which a seller uses economic power in a given area either singularly or jointly to control a market. Actions for monopoly, however, can be brought against buyers as well as sellers. The term *monopsony* refers to a situation where a buyer can reduce competition through purchasing power.[10] It is a challenge of monopsony that is raised against corporations or union trust funds who use their health care purchasing power coercively to dictate prices, exclude recalcitrant sellers, and so reduce competition.[11]

A distinction must be made between the use of business skill to secure favorable pricing arrangements, on the one hand, and the use of economic power in a coercive fashion to control a market and reduce competition, on the other. In the recent federal case, *Royal Drug Co., Inc. v. Group Life and Health Insurance Co.*,[12] the court found that a Blue Shield prescription drug plan that gave preferential reimbursement to participating pharmacies was violative of antitrust law as a monopolistic arrangement. In contrast, the court in *Travelers v. Blue Cross of Western Pennsylvania*[13] did not feel that a special payment

---

*Now the United Mine Workers of America Health and Retirement Funds, as in chapter 12—(ed.).

OVERVIEW OF ANTITRUST LAW

Antitrust law is designed to control the exercise of private economic power by fostering open and fair competition. This body of law grew out of the "common law" where violations for restraint of trade, monopoly, business conspiracy, etc. all had their origins. The "common law" however, proved to be an inadequate vehicle for business regulation and thus as early as the turn of the century the thrust of antitrust enforcement has been statutory. On both the federal and state level statutes and the judicial interpretation of them define the parameters of acceptable competitive behavior.

The following is a list of the major federal antitrust statutes with key provisions highlighted:

Sherman Act (15USC§1-7) Section 1 makes unlawful "every contract, combination . . . or restraint of trade in interstate or foreign commerce." Section 2 prohibits monopolizing, attempts to monopolize and combinations or conspiracies to monopolize any part of interstate or foreign commerce.

Clayton Act (15USC§§12-27) Section 3 prohibits sales on conditions that the buyer not deal with competitors of the seller (i.e. tie-in sales, exclusive dealing arrangements). Section 4 allows private parties injured by violations of the Sherman and Clayton Acts to sue for treble damages. Section 6 exempts labor unions and agricultural organizations from the Sherman and Clayton Acts. Section 7 prohibits acquisitions or mergers where the effect "may be substantially to lessen competition or tend to create a monopoly in any line of commerce in any section of the country." Section 8 prohibits any person from being a director of two or more competing corporations.

Federal Trade Commission Act (15USC§§41-51) Section 5(a)(1) prohibits "unfair methods of competition in commerce and unfair or deceptive acts or practices in commerce." This Act created the Federal Trade Commission (FTC), an administrative agency with broad powers to enforce the antitrust laws.

Robinson–Patman Act (15USC§13) amends the Clayton Act, making it unlawful for any person engaged in commerce to discriminate in price between different purchasers of commodities of like grade and quality where the effect may be to substantially lessen competition or to create a monopoly. Both the seller who offers and the preferred buyer who knowingly receives discriminating prices are guilty of violating the act.

McCarran–Ferguson Act (15USC§1011) provides that federal antitrust laws are applicable to the business of insurance but only to the extent that business is not regulated by state law. However, state regulation cannot render lawful any act or agreement to boycott, coerce or intimidate; such actions would be considered violations of federal law.

Cellar–Kefauver Act amended Section 7 of the Clayton Act to make unlawful the acquisition, by any corporation subject to FTC jurisdiction, of "the stock or any part of the assets of another corporation also engaged in commerce" where the effect of the acquisition may be "to substantially lessen competition in any line of commerce in any section of the country."

The following is a broad categorization of the types of violations the antitrust law is designed to deal with.

1. Horizontal Restraints. A primary purpose of antitrust law has been to preserve and encourage competition among firms in the same industry. Collaboration among competing firms is often referred to as a horizontal restraint; such behavior falls within Section 1 of the Sherman Act.

2. Vertical Restraints. Antitrust law prohibits anticompetitive arrangements between sellers (manufacturers) and buyers (retailers) which could be designed to set prices, limit distribution, etc.; such tie-in arrangements in the various stages of production, distribution of an item are often referred to as vertical restraints. Vertical restraints may constitute violations of Sections 1 and 2 of the Sherman Act and Section 3 of the Clayton Act.

3. Monopolization. Monopoly is the use of market power to control prices or exclude competition in the relevant market. The illegal use of purchasing power to control a given market is referred to as monopsony. Monopoly violations generally fall under Section two of the Sherman Act.

4. Mergers and Acquisitions. A very difficult problem in antitrust law is whether market structure alone can be illegal, for instance, are antitrust laws violated if a firm grows so large (through merger acquisition) that it has the power to restrain competition by its size alone? Under Section 7 of the Clayton Act the government has the power to enjoin corporate mergers that seriously jeopardize competition.

5. Price Discrimination. Sellers who discriminate in prices between purchasers and thus lessen competition by so doing are in violation of the Robinson Patman Act.

6. Unfair Methods of Competition. Business practices which are designed to stifle competition by use of a dominant market position are apt to be classified as unfair methods of competition, particularly when they do not fit under a specific violation of the Clayton or Sherman Act. Unfair competition falls under the Federal Trade Commission Act as well as unfair and deceptive practices in commerce such as false or misleading advertisement.

It should be noted that states have similar antitrust laws that in many instances parallel the federal statutes designed to cover intrastate violations. Finally the reader must be aware of the fact that antitrust law is a fluid area shaped by frequent changes in judicial interpretation and legislative amendments to the law. Presently on the federal level there is a major effort geared toward review and amendment of antitrust laws. Statutory immunities that protect particular industries (e.g., McCarran–Ferguson, insurance) could well be abolished in favor of more extensive antitrust law enforcement.

arrangement Blue Cross had with area hospitals was coercive or constituted an illegal use of monopsony power. In *Travelers* the court reasoned that the defendant's preferential reimbursement scheme was the result of sound business practices, and while it gave Blue Cross a stronger market position, it did not destroy competition. In both *Royal Drug* and *Travelers* the insurers held significant market power, but in the former case the court was convinced that the power was the result of anticompetitive practices.

Multiple Employer Arrangements

Antitrust challenges will not be limited to situations involving one large corporation; they could just as easily be brought against groups of employers who use their economic power to restrain trade in the medical marketplace. The number of corporations who possess adequate purchasing power for antitrust purposes in a given health market is in fact rather small. It is more likely that antitrust challenges, if they emerge, will be brought against groups of employers whose use of joint purchasing power is claimed to go beyond a health purchasing consortium to actually stifling competition in a particular area.

An example of a powerful health purchasing group is the Michigan United Auto Workers' hearing aid benefits plan, which includes the labor union, Ford Motor Company, the Chrysler Corporation, and General Motors. The plan—the first major union program of its kind—covers the full cost of audiometric testing, hearing aid evaluation, and the hearing aid itself. It was implemented in October 1977 through Blue Cross and covers 6 million people. Health professionals to be paid under the plan must agree to participate—that is, accept whatever the insurer decides is appropriate as full compensation. Those who do not so agree cannot receive reimbursement under the plan, and the patient must pay them out of pocket. Currently, the plan's legality is being challenged by two Michigan otolaryngologists, partly on the grounds that it constitutes an illegal restraint of trade in the form of price fixing.[14]

McCarran-Ferguson

The McCarran-Ferguson Act exempts insurers from coverage under the Sherman Antitrust Act to the extent they are covered by state law.[15] Corporate health managers should consider its impact on proposed joint arrangements with insurers and on corporate health plans that have the characteristics of insurance plans.

It should be noted that regulation under state law does not have to deal with the specific insurance practice under challenge; a general state regulatory scheme governing insurance practices will be sufficient for purposes of the McCarran-Ferguson Act.[16] Also, the act is not an absolute bar to federal antitrust coverage because conduct that constitutes an unreasonable restraint of trade through boycott, coercion, or intimidation is not protected. In assessing the effects of McCarran-Ferguson on agreements between insurers and corporations to reduce health care costs, one must consider first whether such arrangements constitute the "business of insurance" and thus come within the McCarran-Ferguson Act. If they do, one must then consider what constitutes a restraint of trade in these arrangements such that the exception provision of McCarran-Ferguson is applicable.

Two cases decided in federal courts have resulted in controversy over the meaning of the "business of insurance." In *Manasen v. California Dental Services*[17] an antitrust challenge was brought by eleven dentists against a prepaid dental care plan. Dentists participating in the plan were required to conform to a usual, customary, and reasonable fee schedule and to accept the plan reimbursement as full payment. Full benefits were paid only to participating dentists, a provision that discouraged enrollees from using nonparticipating practitioners. The plaintiffs contended that the arrangement constituted a conspiracy under federal law to fix dental fees by boycotting dentists who refused to participate and further constituted a monopoly of prepaid dental care in the state of California. They argued that the plan in question did not constitute the "business of insurance" because it was not licensed by the state department of insurance but rather was governed by a California health services plan statute. The Ninth Circuit District Court, however, held that the McCarran-Ferguson exemption was not limited to insurance companies but covered the range of activities affecting rate making, including settlement of claims and limitation of cost. The prepaid plan's role in setting the level of dental fees was recognized by the court as being within the "business of insurance" because it was a key factor in determining the cost of premiums. It was thus found exempt from federal regulation.

In direct conflict with the decision in *Manasen* is the case of *Royal Drug Co., Inc. v. Group Life and Health Insurance Co.*[18] In *Royal Drug* a number of independent pharmacies challenged on antitrust grounds a Blue Shield plan under which insured beneficiaries were required to pay only two dollars for prescriptions purchased from participating pharmacies. In nonparticipating pharmacies, the insured had to pay the full prescription price and were later reimbursed 75 percent of the costs exceeding the two-dollar deductible. The plaintiff pharmacies argued that the plan constituted price fixing, an unlawful restraint of trade, and also encouraged an insured to boycott nonparticipating pharmacies. The Fifth Circuit Court of Appeals found that the relationship between the insurance carrier and the participating pharmacies concerning prices did not involve the insured and as such did not come within the "business of insurance." In taking direct aim on the *Manasen* decision, the court stated that "an activity is not part of the business of insurance solely because it has an impact, favorable or otherwise, upon premiums charged by the insurer." One hopes that this dispute in the federal court decisions will ultimately be resolved by the Supreme Court, but the weight is clearly on the broader view of the "business of insurance" taken by the Ninth Circuit in *Manasen*.[19]

The analogies are strong between these carrier-provider cases and the care providers. It can be argued that such arrangements, whether they be agreements to abide by a fee schedule, a second opinion program, or utilization review, affect the cost of the premium for the corporate buyer (and of the insured where employee contribution is required) and as such fall within the McCarran-Ferguson "business of insurance" definition. In fact, almost any element in a corporate health plan insurance arrangement with providers can be considered to be in the "business of insurance," thus placing the arrangement under the McCarran-Ferguson Act.

Once it has been determined that a particular corporation-insurance company arrangement is covered by McCarran-Ferguson, the question arises whether the exception provision of the statute is applicable. Use of the exception provision had also been the subject of dispute among federal courts, but the Supreme Court in *St. Paul Fire and Marine Insurance Co. v. Barry*[20] ended the controversy when it upheld a lower court decision that the McCarran-Ferguson exception was intended to be read broadly. According to the Supreme Court, the exception provision covers any act or agreement amounting to a boycott, coercion, or intimidation.

This leaves the issue of what constitutes a boycott, coercion, or intimidation under the McCarran-Ferguson Act. In *Travelers v. Blue Cross of Western Pennsylvania*[21] the plaintiff accused the defendant insurance company of coercive practices in its dealings with hospitals. The court rejected the argument, finding that the hospital contracts were not a form of coercion but were agreements jointly negotiated and approved by the state insurance department. The court ruled that McCarran-Ferguson was applicable, thereby removing the action from the Sherman Act, but also proceeded to dispell, for the sake of argument, the applicability of restraint of trade challenge. The court reasoned that Blue Cross practices in negotiating lower rates with hospitals were in the interest of good business, a valid means of reducing costs.

In *Proctor v. State Farm Insurance Co.*[22] the District of Columbia Court of Appeals engaged in an extensive discussion of the McCarran-Ferguson boycott exception. While the court agreed that the exception should be applied broadly, it did not feel that a preferred payment arrangement for certain auto repair shops constituted a boycott of nonpreferred shops. The court in *Proctor* went so far as to acknowledge that the arrangements in question could be classified as a "collective refusal to deal," but may still not be a boycott: "so long as policyholders are not prevented from utilizing nonpreferred shops, the degree of coercive enforcement activity required to convert mere cooperation or concert of action into boycott, coercion, or intimidation is not present."

From an evaluation of the case law it seems that for the McCarran-Ferguson exception to apply, corporate-insurer agreements would have to severely restrict the insured beneficiaries' freedom of choice, that is, the insured workers world have to be *prevented* from going to nonparticipating providers. The case law does not recognize a discrepancy in indemnity arrangements among providers offered by a given plan as constituting boycott, coercion, or intimidation.

What Law Governs Self-Funded Plans?

Those employers who choose to go beyond insurance company cost intervention schemes and establish self-funded plans to cover health benefits (either alone or in a multiple employer arrangement) must weigh a number of legal considerations. They must assess the potential effects of the Employee Retirement Income Security Act of 1974 (ERISA), with its detailed reporting and fiduciary requirements.[23] They must also be aware of tax law because self-funding arrangements qualify as 501(c)(9) trusts under the Internal Revenue Code and as such are eligible for a number of tax advantages, but such status is not without its limitations.[24] The most common legal consideration in regard to self-funding arises from the corporation's role as it replaces the insurance carrier. Contractual arrangements developed with providers will be subject to state law. Also, the corporation must deal directly with claims, which may significantly add to legal costs.[25]

A key issue in decisions of whether to self-fund and how to structure a given plan is the question of what law applies to a health benefit plan: the federal law (ERISA) or the respective state insurance statutes?

Under the constitutional doctrine of supremacy, if a clash occurs between federal and state law, federal law supercedes.[26] ERISA contains a seemingly clear-cut federal preemption in section 514, which specifies that all state laws dealing with employee benefit plans are preempted by federal law. The preemption is modified in section 514(b)(2)(A) by a "savings clause" which allows states to continue to exercise regulatory authority over the "business of insurance," but states cannot classify employee benefit plans as insurance, according to what is referred to as the "deemer clause" in section 514(b)(2)(B). The override of state regulation under ERISA has stimulated interest in self-funding because it abolishes dual jurisdictional requirements and permits multistate plan uniformity.[27] The section 514 preemption has been generally—but not always—upheld: there are situations where state insurance regulations are not totally precluded from covering employee health benefit plans, particularly when they involve multiple employer trusts.

Section 514 Exemption

A number of state attorneys general have addressed the issue of preemption under section 514 of ERISA and have strongly supported the supremacy of federal law. For example, the Oklahoma attorney general took the position that self-insured health benefit plans should be considered employee welfare benefit plans under ERISA, and as such, be preempted from state law.[28] The New York state attorney general held that employees' beneficiary associations under section 501(c)(9) of the Internal Revenue Code are not subject to licensing and regulatory authority under the state insurance laws.[29] The Idaho attorney general ruled that an Idaho law providing for the registration and supervision of self-funded health care plans was preempted by ERISA.[30]

In the case law the strongest endorsement of preemption under ERISA occurs in the Ninth Circuit District Court opinion of *Hewlett-Packard v. Barnes*.[30] At issue here was the scope of California's Knox-Keene law, under which all health care service plans were subject to the regulation of the California Commissioner of Corporations. The court examined the legislative history of section 514 of ERISA[31] which proved to be strongly in favor of the broad application of federal law. According to Senator Harrison Williams, chairman of the Senate Committee on Labor and Public Welfare (as quoted by the court), "it should be stressed that with the narrow exceptions specified in the bill the substantive and enforcement provisions are intended to preempt the field for federal regulations, thus eliminating the threat of conflicting or inconsistent state and local regulations of employee benefit plans." The defendant state of California argued that Knox-Keene applied because under ERISA states retain the right to regulate insurance, and health care service plans are a form of insurance. The court rejected this contention as being in clear conflict with the "deemer" clause of ERISA.[32]

The case of *Insurer's Action Council, Inc. v. Heaton*[33] was the first federal court action in which a more restrictive approach toward preemption under ERISA was adopted. A group of insurers sought to enjoin the enforcement of the Minnesota Comprehensive Insurance Act of 1976, a part of which required employers who offer health benefit plans to provide certain types of state-qualified plans. They argued that the state statutory benefit plan requirements were preempted by ERISA. The court rejected the preemption argument, holding that ERISA overrides only the reporting and disclosure requirements of state health and accident insurance laws. What was at issue in *Insurer's Action Council* were neither reporting nor disclosure requirements, but rather the substance of insurance plans, and this, according to the court, was a matter of state law because ERISA did not preempt state insurance regulation.

Insurer's Action Council raises the issue of the relationship between the ERISA preemption and the McCarran-Ferguson Act. According to McCarran-

Ferguson, the regulation of insurance is to be left to the states, and this right of state regulatory power is recognized in ERISA section 514(b)(2)(A). The basic question here is whether an employee health benefit plan constitutes insurance. ERISA precludes a state from deeming that a given benefit plan is insurance, as can be seen in *Hewlett-Packard.* On the other hand, by interpreting the preemption doctrine narrowly the court in *Insurer's Action Council* decided that only certain activities come within ERISA's federal override provision, thus increasing the states' role in regulating employee benefit plans (seemingly more in keeping with the McCarran-Ferguson Act).[34]

The issue in *Wadsworth v. Whaland,*[35] a recent federal court case, was whether New Hampshire could impose a unique state law detailing special requirements for employee health benefit plans. The statute in question required that carriers of group health insurance provide coverage for treatment of mental illness and emotional disorders. The administrators of several health and welfare funds sought to overturn the law. The particular funds involved were self-insured for a few benefits, but almost 90 percent of their benefits were provided through group insurance policies. The plaintiffs argued that section 514 of ERISA preempts any indirect or direct regulation of employee benefit plans by state government, and that while the statute in question dealt with the contents of group insurance policies, it affected employee benefit plans by increasing their premium costs. The *Wadsworth* court ruled that the New Hampshire law was exempted from ERISA preemption by virtue of section 514(b)(2)(A) of the federal law. The court recognized the fact that a state may not classify an employee benefits plan as insurance but found nothing within ERISA that prohibited a state from indirectly affecting plans by regulating the contents of the group insurance policies they purchased. This decision has recently been upheld by the United States Supreme Court.

Multiple Employer Trusts

Considerable debate exists over the effect of the ERISA section 514 exemption on multiple employer trusts (MET). A MET is usually a nonprofit 501(c)(9) self-funded employee benefits plan financed by a group of employers (see chapter 4). With the failure of some MET plans, interest has grown in removing them from ERISA protection to allow state regulatory control, or in establishing federal guidelines in this area.[36] An activities report of the Committee on Education and Labor of the United States House of Representatives expressed concern over the marketing of insurance products by certain entrepreneurs as ERISA-covered plans. The Department of Labor has not developed a unified policy concerning the relationship of ERISA and METs largely because of the diversity in the way METs are structured. Recently, the Department of Labor did issue guidelines to be used in interpreting whether a MET falls under ERISA coverage.[37]

The question whether a given MET plan falls under ERISA has been addressed by several federal courts. The United States District Court for the District of Kansas in *Bell v. Employee Security Benefit Association*[38] was confronted with determining whether an association that engaged in direct solicitation of employees and purported to be an employee organization came under the ERISA preemption. The defendant Employee Security Benefit Association (ESBA) was advertised as a self-funded, self-adjusting employee benefit plan under ERISA. The *Bell* court identified two legal issues to be dealt with: the scope of preemption and the question whether ESBA was insurance or a self-funded plan. The court came down strongly in favor of a broad preemption under ERISA, citing a recent House Committee Report that stated there was congressional intent to ensure uniformity of regulation by precluding state authority over plans. On the second issue, ESBA as insurance or self-funded plan, the court came down on the side of insurance. "Our conclusion is that just as a state cannot regulate an employee benefit plan by calling it insurance, neither can defendants merchandise an insurance program free of state regulation by terming it an employee benefit plan."[39] The court recognized that employee welfare plans have many insurance elements, but the test adopted to determine whether the plan in question constituted insurance confirmed that ESBA was a form of insurance and not a welfare benefits plan. The court was influenced in its decision by the facts that the plan was not established and maintained by an employer or a preexisting employee group it was provided by a third-party entrepreneur with a profit motive and sold on the basis of its actuarial soundness.[40]

The problems that have arisen in effectively regulating METs have led to proposed amendments to ERISA. Recently introduced Senate Bill No. 3017, proposes significant changes in the original ERISA statute, including provisions for regulating METs in a fashion similar to other ERISA-qualified plans.[41]

Confidentiality of Employee Medical Records

Corporations attempting to reduce the cost of employee health benefits need detailed information about their employees' health status. Company medical departments typically possess considerable data, but they have no way of finding out the nature of claims filed by a given employee with the insurance carrier. Some companies contemplating self-funding have sought access to employee insurance records in order to assess the types of services their health care expenditures were purchasing.[42]

This need for more detailed medical information is only the initial information problem. The more difficult issue is how corporations will handle the increasing flow of employee health data that is bound to result when they become more involved in controlling medical expenditures. The issue of the rights of employees' confidentiality of medical records will become of key importance to corporate health benefit managers and medical departments.

Currently, the issue of confidentiality of medical data has been eclipsed by a desire on the part of workers and unions to expand the health benefits package. Still, the confidentiality issue has recently been the subject of controversy in the corporate sector. For example, the refusal of DuPont workers to consent to the release of health records resulted in a lawsuit against DuPont by the National Institute of Occupational Safety and Health.[43] With a significant increase in the amount of personal medical information corporations collect, the level of interest in safeguarding that information from misuse is likely to increase.

The law dealing with medical records offers few protections of a physician-patient privilege and some limited statutory safeguards. Perhaps the employer-employee relationship will expand to where medical privacy will be safeguarded under the rubric of that relationship, but at present this is not the case. In corporations that have developed medical confidentiality policies, a worker may be able to uphold his or her rights under a contractual agreement or in a union setting under collective bargaining. By and large, however, the protection of workers' medical files is solely a matter of corporate policy. It has been suggested that a federal statute similar to the Privacy Act be passed to regulate the activities of the private sector in the record-keeping area.[44]

The increase in health care data held by the corporation will necessitate the development of medical confidentiality policies. The New York Telephone Company has outlined four fundamental principles for medical privacy:

> "(1) A conceptual difference must be accepted between (a) medical informa-
> tion and (b) conclusions or judgments with the former receiving a higher
> degree of protection; (2) confidentiality of medical information must be
> absolute and uniform; (3) determination of what information is to be kept
> confidential and what may be released is the prerogative of the patient
> employee, not of the corporate medical department; and (4) confidentiality
> is not synonymous with abdication of responsibility on the part of the
> professional."[45]

Corporate medical privacy policies can serve as a guide to management and assist in improving employer-employee relationships, but the law does not allow for total protection of the employee privacy interest. If a corporation has information about an adverse physical condition of a worker, it may be forced to act on the basis of that information.

For example, in the case of *Coffee v. McDonnell-Douglas*[46] defendant corporation was held liable for failing to take into account the results of a blood test prior to giving the plaintiff his work assignment. The greater the amount of employee medical data a corporation possesses, the more its burden will be to take affirmative action when a given medical file so warrants.[47] The corporation is not just a repository of data; it must use the data in individual employee and companywide decision making. Complete confidentiality of employee medical records is more a desired goal than a possible reality given the legal and business pressures to utilize the collected health data. A corporation must, therefore, strike a balance between guarded use of worker health data and protection of those data from misuse.

Conclusion and Recommendations

The above legal issues represent several major areas of the law that corporations should be fully aware of as they choose to become actively involved in controlling health benefits costs. Clearly, the nature of the problems will vary with the type of arrangements a corporation develops. The chances are that most company plans to reduce health benefits costs will not be extensive enough to raise serious legal difficulties. Active corporate efforts to restructure health benefit packages may, however, encounter some of the legal hurdles discussed here.

Several recommendations can be made to assist corporate managers in avoiding these legal problems:

> Prior to working out a cost intervention scheme, corporations should, for antitrust purposes, carefully assess their purchasing power in a given health market. Those corporations with significant purchasing power must be careful not to structure cost control schemes in a fashion that could be deemed to constitute a restraint of trade.

> Corporate schemes to reduce health care costs should be formulated with input from area practitioners. In dealing with the issue of medical fees, corporations must be careful not to accept set fee schedules which could well be struck down as violative of antitrust law.

> While the "business of insurance" clause under the McCarran-Ferguson Act should be read broadly to include a wide range of activities, corporate managers should be aware that antitrust law is a fluid area, and there is currently an ongoing evaluation of federal law in the area that could well lead to repeal of statutory immunities such as that offered in McCarran-Ferguson.

> Finally, while it is essential that corporations be aware of the effects of antitrust law and ERISA on their efforts to establish alternative corporate health plans, neither area should be viewed as presenting insurmountable obstacles to formulating creative, cost effective employee health benefit packages.

The author acknowledges with gratitude the advice of Dr. William J. Bicknell in the preparation of this paper.

NOTES

1. 15 USC §§ 1–7.

2. 15 USC §§ 12–27.

3. 15 USC §§ 41–51.

4. Lawrence A. Sullivan, *Antitrust*, chap. 3, "Horizontal Restraints of Trade," pp. 186–189.

5. Ibid, pp. 196–197. A successful monopoly challenge which demonstrates that the defendants control prices and/or exclude competition is contingent on their having considerable market power.

6. Legal actions in the medical price-fixing area have focused on physician organizations that issue price guidelines to their competitor members. See Remarks of Jonathan E. Gaines, Assistant Director, Bureau of Competition, Federal Trade Commission, before the

Professional Associations Council of the American Society of Association Executives, Washington, D.C., February 10, 1978.

7. Restraint of trade can be achieved in other arrangements besides fee schedules; utilization review or second opinion programs, for example, may adversely affect competition.

8. *Webster County Memorial Hospital, Inc. v. United Mine Workers of America Welfare and Retirement Fund* 536 F2d 419 (1976).

9. Sullivan, *Antitrust*, chap. 1.

10. Ibid., pp. 30–35.

11. It is interesting to note that the hospital in *Webster* never raised the issue of monopsony which may have proven to be a more persuasive argument than restraint of trade.

12. 415 F. Supp. 343 (1976).

13. 481 F2d 80 (1973).

14. *Newsletter of the American Council of Otolaryngology*, vol. 9, no. 6 (December 1977). In any joint or single corporate health plan a key legal consideration will be the development of contractual arrangements. It is important that companies develop contracts with providers that allow sufficient flexibility in cost control efforts. It is further important that corporate-provider agreements are drawn in such a fashion that they cannot be classified as adhesion contracts.

15. 15 USC §§ 1011–1015.

16. See *McIlhinney v. American Title Insurance Co.* 418 F. Supp. 364 (1977).

17. 424 F. Supp. 657 (1976).

18. 415 F. Supp. 343 (1976).

19. Indeed, the majority of federal courts have refused to deny the application of McCarran-Ferguson to professional service plans because they involve the delivery of products and services rather than indemnity. Case precedent and legislative history both seem to indicate that activities constituting the "business of insurance" under McCarran-Ferguson are broader than what constitutes insurance under state law.

20. 46 L.W. 4971 (1978).

21. 481 F2d 80 (1973).

22. 561 F2d 262 (1977).

23. C. B. Renfrew, "Fiduciary Responsibilities under the Pension Reform Act," *Business Law*, vol. 32, p. 1829 (July 1977).

24. Jeffrey Fuller, "The Use of Self-Funded Plans: The Emerging Principles for Affiliated Corporations, Trade Associations and METs," "Discussion of Certain Tax Problems Presented by Self-Funded Employee Welfare Benefit Plans," Practicing Law Institute Eighth Annual Employee Benefit Institute, New York, April 1978, pp. 306–307.

25. Robert E. Kelly, "Self-Funding Welfare Plans, or, There Is No Insurance in Group Insurance," *Proceedings of the 1976 Annual Educational Conference*, International Foundation of Employee Benefit Plans, vol. 18.

26. See *Florida Lime and Avocado Growers, Inc. v. Paul* 373 U.S. 132 (1963); *Rice v. Santa Fe Elevator Corp.* 331 U.S. 218 (1974).

27. Kelly, "No Insurance in Group Insurance."

28. Fuller, "Certain Tax Problem," p. 280.

29. Ibid.

30. Ibid.

31. 425 F. Supp. 1294 (1977).

32. In a similar action in *Azzaro v. Harnett* (515 F. Supp. 473 [1976]), plaintiffs Bakery Drivers Local No. 802 Pension Fund challenged the right of the New York State Division of Insurance to inquire into the benefit status of a pension fund participant. The court

supported the plaintiffs' preemption argument, reasoning that ERISA offers a full range of protection under federal law and thus makes state regulation unnecessary. Regarding the specific state inquiry, the court noted that ERISA requires the administrator of an employee pension benefit plan to furnish any participant a statement of his current status. According to the *Azzaro* court the role of the state in regulating employee welfare plans should be limited to dealing only with those problem areas still existing that predate the implementation of ERISA.

33. 432 F. Supp. 921 (1976).

34. It should be noted, however, that some legal commentators have interpreted *Insurer's Action Council* to hold that ERISA does not preempt state laws regulating insurance as applied to insurers only.

35. 46 L.W. 2155 (1978).

36. United States Senate Bill No. 3017, introduced May 1, 1978.

37. Fuller, "Emerging Principles."

38. 437 F. Supp. 382 (1977).

39. See *Hewlett-Packard v. Barnes*, 425 F. Supp. 1294 (1977).

40. In an action similar to Bell, *Hemberlin v. V.I.P. Insurance Trust* (434 F. Supp. 1196 [1977]), the beneficiaries of a group health and accident policy brought suit alleging violations of ERISA. The legal issue that underlay the action was whether the federal court had subject matter jurisdiction, given that it was questionable whether the plan at issue was covered by ERISA. The insurer of the original V.I.P. Trust, a multiple employer trust, canceled its group coverage, at which point defendant insurance brokers set up a self-funded plan with themselves acting as administrators at a 15 percent commission. The trust was run as a business enterprise of the insurance brokers with employers having no voice in its management, operation, or decisions to terminate; no employer contributions were made on behalf of employees. According to the court, "this trust [V.I.P. Trust] was purely an entrepreneurial plan put together by Galbraith and Green [insurance brokers] to protect business commissions they would have lost if the trust had not been restructured." The decision continued, "there has been substantial national concern over the increase in the numbers of uninsured multiple employer trusts such as this which have avoided state supervision and failed, leaving sick or injured employees holding any empty bag." The *Hamberlin* court ruled that ERISA could not be used as an umbrella to protect purely commercial plans from state regulation; thus the federal court denied that it had jurisdiction under ERISA to consider the merits of the claim.

41. S. 3017 also exempts the interest of an employee in an employee benefit plan from being characterized as a security under the Securities and Exchange Act, another area of jurisdictional controversy. It should also be noted that HMOs, according to the Department of Labor (Press Release 77-188), are to be classified as benefits and not employee benefit plans subject to ERISA. The Labor Department opinion has been supported in the Ninth Circuit opinion of *Hewlett-Packard v. Barnes* (425 F. Supp. 1294 [1977]).

42. Some insurance companies have refused to grant corporations permission to examine identified employee health insurance records. While part of the reason for the refusal is concern for confidentiality, a more practical consideration is the cost to the insurer of assembling the data.

43. *DuPont v. Finklea* S.D.W.V. December 20, 1977, No. 88–2059.

44. Fred J. Gregura, "Informational Privacy and the Private Sector," *Creighton Law Review*, vol. 11, p. 312 (1977).

45. G. H. Collings, "Medical Confidentiality in the Work Environment," in *The Civil Liberties Review Individual Rights Sourcebook*, vol. II, Alan Westin ed. (New York: ACLU 1978), p. 276.

46. 503 P. 2d 1366 (1972).

47. John D. Blum, "Corporate Liability for Inhouse Medical Malpractice," *St. Louis University Law Journal*, vol. 22 (Summer 1978).

Appendix

Conference Participants Quoted*

John L. Bauer, Jr., Supervisor, Insurance Benefits, Armco Corporation, Middletown, Ohio

William J. Bicknell, M.D., M.P.H., Director, Special Health Programs, Boston University and Medical Director, United Mine Workers of America Health and Retirement Funds, Boston, Massachusetts and Washington, D.C.

Jack H. Bleuler, Health Benefits Advisor, Mobil Oil Corporation, New York, New York

James H. Brennan, Jr., Vice President, Towers, Perrin, Forster and Crosby, New York, New York

John L. Brown, Director, Employee Benefits, Genesco, Inc., Nashville, Tennessee

Arthur G. Carty, President, Blue Cross of Massachusetts, Inc., Boston, Massachusetts

Stephen C. Caulfield, Assistant Director for Regional Operations, United Mine Workers of America Health and Retirement Funds, Washington, D.C.

Henry A. DiPrete, Second Vice President, Group Operations, John Hancock Mutual Life Insurance Co., Boston, Massachusetts

Robert F. Froehlke, President, Health Insurance Association of America, Washington, D.C.

*Including authors of background papers

Willis B. Goldbeck, Director, Washington Business Group on Health, Washington, D.C.

Galt Grant, Manager, Corporate Insurance Administration, Polaroid Corporation, Cambridge, Massachusetts

Michael J. Gulotta, Actuarial Assistant, American Telephone and Telegraph Company, Piscataway, New Jersey

Donald P. Harrington, Director, Benefits Planning and Analysis, American Telephone and Telegraph Company, Basking Ridge, New Jersey

Geoffrey V. Heller, Consultant-Health Legislation, University of California, Statewide Administration, Berkeley, California

John Hickey, Partner, Kwasha-Lipton, Consulting Actuaries Division, Englewood Cliffs, New Jersey

Bernard T. Hurley, Jr., Vice President, Industry and Government Relations, Provident Life and Accident Insurance Company, Chattanooga, Tennessee

Samuel X. Kaplan, President, United States Administrators, Los Angeles, California

Brant Kelch, Director of Health Care Financing and Program Development, United Mine Workers of America, Health and Retirement Funds, Washington, D.C.

Michael P. McDonald, Vice President, Marketing, Blue Cross-Blue Shield Associations, Chicago, Illinois

William Michelson, President, United Storeworkers Security Plan, New York, New York

Judith K. Miller, Director, National Health Policy Forum, George Washington University, Washington, D.C.

Joseph W. Mullen, Jr., Vice President, Group Insurance and Pensions, Metropolitan Life Insurance Company, New York, NY

Gordon W. Thomas, Vice President, Group Operations, John Hancock Mutual Life Insurance Company, Boston, Massachusetts

Gilbert S. Omenn, M.D., Ph.D., Assistant Director for Human Resources and Social and Economic Services, Executive Office of the President, Office of Science and Technology Policy, Washington, D.C.

Robert B. Peters, Manager, Compensation and Benefits, Mobil Oil Corporation, New York, New York

Harvey Pies, Assistant Minority Counsel, Committee on Ways and Means, House of Representatives, Washington, D.C.

Robert B. Poitras, President, Tamarack Management Corporation, Pembroke, Massachusetts

Thomas O. Pyle, Executive Vice President, Harvard Community Health Plan, Allston, Massachusetts

Lesley L. Ralson, Senior Vice President, Group Insurance Department, The Prudential Insurance Company of America, Newark, New Jersey

Albert F. Ritardi, Director, Administration and Medical Services, Allied Chemical Corporation, Morristown, New Jersey

Steven Sieverts, Vice President for Institutional Affairs and Health Care Cost Containment, Blue Cross-Blue Shield of Greater New York, New York, New York

Bruce F. Spencer, Editor, Charles D. Spencer and Associates, Chicago, Illinois

Jacob J. Spies, Assistant Vice President, Division of Health Care Systems, Employers Insurance of Wausau, Wausau, Wisconsin

Kevin Stokeld, Manager, Health Care Planning, Deere and Company, Moline, Illinois

Richard W. Stone, M.D., Medical Director, Research, American Telephone and Telegraph Company, Basking Ridge, New Jersey

Timothy B. Sullivan, Vice President, Administration, L. G. Balfour Company, Attleboro, Massachusetts

Kenneth A. Tannenbaum, D.D.S., President, Health Systems Group, Inc., Ann Arbor, Michigan

Gordon W. Thomas, Senior Vice President, Group Insurance Operations, John Hancock Mutual Life Insurance Company, Boston, Massachusetts

Eleanor J. Tilson, Administrator, United Storeworkers Security Plan, New York, New York

David C. Wineland, Manager, Employee Benefits, Armco Corporation, Middletown, Ohio

David H. Winkworth, Manager, Insurance and Legislated Benefits Section, Mobil Oil Corporation, New York, New York